The Emotional Journey To Successful Weight Loss

Daryl Marceau

To Shaula and Gary,
Thanks again for all
your help in making my
book a reality. I can't
say enough.

Disclaimer: The information in this book is for entertainment purposes only and does not constitute health advice in any way. The author, Daryl Marceau, is not a doctor or health practitioner. The reader is advised to consult with your health practitioner before embarking on any weight loss or exercise program.

Published by Prominence Publishing. www.prominencepublishing.com

ISBN: 978-0-9958274-0-0

First Edition: December 2016

I dedicate this book to my loving wife. You continue to see in me what I didn't always see in myself. Your support is why this book was written and for that I am forever grateful.

PREFACE

As I sat talking with my old friend Craig, I began describing the different feelings and emotions I was having about my life. I stated that it felt so unfair that I had to go through so much for so many years in my struggle with my weight. I spoke about being bullied as a child and the self hatred I experienced as an adult. But I also spoke of the positive change that has occurred within me over the last 11 months as I lost 155 pounds. I shared that I was feeling really good about myself and excited about what was next in my life. I told Craig about my plan to write a book about the emotional journey to weight loss. I had come to believe that healing one's spirit, heart and mind had to happen before any true lasting change could occur. I went on to say that this was especially true with weight loss. I explained that, although I was excited about sharing my experiences and thoughts, I was still struggling with something on the inside. I was finding it really difficult to find meaning in my often difficult past.

Craig looked at me and said that maybe I was meant to go through what I did. I looked at him a little funny and he went on to explain that not everyone had my strength or knew how to tap into their inner power. Craig had my full attention as he discussed the possibility that all my struggles were meant to prepare me for something greater. I had presence and an ability to help people see their potential. In that moment Craig helped me realize that everything that had happened up until today was needed so that I could help others heal and change their lives. The difficult days could also be seen as training days to prepare me for what I was about to do. My past was not something to reject but something to be grateful for. Without all the experiences over the last 43 years, this book would likely not have been written. I wasn't being punished. I was being chosen for something greater. I always knew deep inside that I would one day help a lot of people and now the opportunity had presented itself. Over the last year I have been on an emotional journey that changed my life and now I am excited to share it with you. I believe that everyone has the ability to live the life they want. They just need to know how to get there. This goes for weight loss too. So, if you're willing to take the first step on the path to successful, long lasting weight loss then turn the page and let's go....

Table of Contents

Preface v

Introduction 1

Chapter 1: Am I Ready? 5

Chapter 2: Assembling Your Support Team............................. 10

Chapter 3: Preparing for your Emotional Journey 13

　　My Story.. 16

　　Your Story. 23

Chapter 4: Identifying Your Themes and Patterns 27

Chapter 5: Picking Your Start Date....................................... 34

Chapter 6: Preparing for Challenges 37

Chapter 7: Specific Goal Setting.. 40

Chapter 8: Preparing for DAY 1.. 45

　　Eating Plan 47

　　Exercise Plan... 52

　　The Gym.. 55

　　Emotional and Psychological Preparation 57

Chapter 9: Getting Started.. 62

　　Week 1 64

　　Week 2 67

　　Week 3 68

　　Week 4 70

Chapter 10: Hitting Your Stride 73

Weeks 5-8 73

Week 9-16 76

Weeks 17-25 79

Chapter 11: Going the Distance 83

Week 26-52 83

Chapter 12: Getting Real Once and For All – The Final
Commitment 88

Chapter 13: Weight Issues And Relationships 93

Chapter 14: Weight Loss Issues and Children 96

Chapter 15: Alternative Weight Loss Options (Surgery) 99

Conclusion 104

Acknowledgements 109

Appendix 1 111

Eating Plan Ideas 111

Appendix 2 114

Keep in Touch 116

Introduction

I would like to start by thanking you for purchasing this book. This book is different than most weight loss books out there. It is written by someone who knows what it is like to be morbidly obese and struggle with the emotional challenges of food addiction. I am not a doctor, nutritionist nor a personal trainer. I am a social worker by trade. Unlike many health professionals, personal trainers, counsellors etc. I have experienced the full range of weight and health, from being morbidly obese at 400+ pounds to being very fit. I get what it's like to feel stuck and through my own experience and research I was able to find a way to lose weight and keep it off. It continues to be an exciting journey of self discovery.

What makes the "The Emotional Journey to Successful Weight Loss" different is that it doesn't just focus on one aspect of weight loss but a range of factors to help you maximize the likelihood that you will lose weight and keep it off. This book is not as much a how-to guide to lose weight as it is a map to support you in your own journey. Included are ideas around healthy eating and exercise but ultimately this book is more than just that. I have learned that the key to weight loss is to first focus on the mental and emotional aspects connected to overeating. By just focusing on one aspect (diet or exercise), you may have limited success, but by putting everything together and using all the resources at your disposal, your chances of losing excess weight and maintaining a healthy weight is much higher.

This book has you look at your own life story as it is connected to food, challenges you to change the unhealthy behaviours connected to emotional eating and then gives you a look into what to expect when embarking on the emotional journey to weightloss. There are lots of extras too including my life story and the impact that food addiction had on it. The book also looks at food journalling, goal setting, how to get started, using the weight scale, making the most of the different resources and supports, going to the gym, an alternative to traditional weight loss, and making the final commitment.

If you are currently struggling with weight or food issues, you will likely relate to many of the same experiences that I'm about to share. We have all tried different diets and weight loss programs. Often we are successful for a period of time but then go back to our old ways, inevitably gaining back the weight and sometimes more. We then struggle to get back on track, often beating ourselves up along the way. I have developed a way to take the weight off and keep it off. I know by taking the steps outlined in this book you too will be able to lose weight and keep it off.

Many people I have talked to about my weight loss journey will start by being really interested in what I have to say. But as I start talking, they often begin to glaze over. I hope it is not because I am boring them. It's likely due to the fact that when I explain there is hard work involved, including doing the emotional work and committing to healthy eating and daily exercise, they no longer want to listen. There is much more to successful weight loss than eating less and working out more. There is no magic pill or simple answer. It is a process that takes time, discipline and a lifelong commitment. I understand the complexity of the emotional and social challenges that obese people struggle with every day. I believe successful, long term weight loss is 95 percent mental. Once you have a good handle on the emotional end of your food and weight issues, then the healthy eating and exercise will fall into place. I won't lie. It's going to take work but the rewards will be lifelong and worthwhile.

I will be with you every step of the way in your weight loss journey. I will give you ideas, share my own experiences and challenge you in supportive ways to stop old patterns of thinking and create new thoughts and behaviours. Everyone holds a wealth of inner knowledge and resources needed to be successful. I will help you unlock your own knowledge and resources to make the changes you desire become reality. I will work with you, not only on healthy eating and exercise, but on what I believe to be the most vital part – the "emotional work" of weight loss. Other books may solely focus on diet and exercise. But what has been missing is how to make the mental and emotional shifts needed to change our relationships with food and exercise. By doing this, we will be able to maintain a healthy lifestyle for the rest of our lives. Once we find a way to change our thinking, coping and behaviours, our lives will change in ways we didn't think imaginable.

So, let's start the journey – the journey to a healthier life where you are in control and can make choices that are right for you. I have lost 155 pounds in 10 months and you too can have the results you desire.

Chapter 1

Am I Ready?

Before you start your journey there are two important questions you need to ask yourself, "Do I really want this?" and "Am I ready?" The reason I ask you this is that this is a big commitment and to be truly successful you will need to both challenge yourself and ask yourself some difficult questions. Many people say they are ready but quit when things get difficult. In the past I have started and given up many times which often sank me deeper into my depression and rut. I want to help you avoid the weight loss - weight gain cycle so many of us have experienced. However, before you do this it's time to have the first big talk with yourself. You will need to ask yourself if you are willing to trust this process and willing to stick it out through the tough times when the desire to eat unhealthy foods or stay on the couch is almost unbearable. If you are ready then let's do this. If you're unsure, then I challenge you to ask yourself both why you are ready and why you aren't as well as what you need to do to be ready. (See the worksheet on page 8 to help you guide your decision).

For me, the moment I knew I was ready was in December of 2014. I was walking through our local mall and felt defeated, sad and depressed. I was nearing 400 pounds again and could only shop in the Big and Tall store. I felt uncomfortable in my clothes and with myself. I lacked energy, optimism and joy. I wasn't being who I knew I could be and it scared me that I would be living another year of my life sad and uninspired. I felt a sense of desperation and a longing to be happy. I wanted to be at a weight where I felt confident and happy in my own skin. I was tired, both physically and emotionally, and although I presented as the funny guy on the outside, on the inside I was dying. I knew somewhere deep inside me that if I didn't do something the chances of sinking deeper into depression and experiencing some type of serious health issue was definitely on the horizon.

New Year's Day was a few days away and I would likely be making the same resolution I did every year. I also knew that I really wanted to be healthy and fit and I was ready to try losing the weight again. However, this time something inside of me said that if I did this I needed to really commit and make it a lifelong change. I was fed up with losing a substantial amount of weight only to gain it back and feel worse about myself. As I walked by and saw my reflection in the mirror (which I didn't really like at the time) I said to myself, "Daryl you need to change and you need to change now. But this time you're doing this in a healthy and long lasting way." I wasn't quite sure what this truly meant at the time but I knew within me something felt a little different. I wasn't just saying it. I really believed that a life change was possible and necessary. I thought about what I needed to do to be ready. I didn't have to do this for long as I was tired of the same old cycle and way of being that was not bringing me the happiness that I desired. I also knew that when I did this I needed to have a plan and be methodical and strategic about it. I needed to bring everything I knew about weight loss (as well as educate myself on things I didn't know) in order to create long lasting results.

If you're struggling with these questions (do I really want this? am I ready?) this may be the time you decide to enlist help. For me, I found a counsellor who challenged me regarding my perfectionism and all or nothing thinking. I spoke about wanting to change but the fear that came with it especially if I failed again. She helped me see that everything leading up to now was part of my journey and learning. My counsellor's support helped me gain further understanding of myself and my relationship with food. The more I spoke with her about my story and how I was feeling, the more I realized that I was ready and this was my time.

I believe that this is your time for change. By buying this book, you are likely getting to the point of being ready to make your move. You're also likely craving change in your life around food, health and happiness. Now you can use this desire and energy to begin taking the steps necessary in your journey.

Below is your first task. Be honest when you fill it out. If you are not honest, you are only deceiving yourself. Ask yourself if you really want this? Why or why not? Then write down the reasons you are ready and the reason you are not. Next, consider the reasons that you are not yet ready for this weight loss journey. Write down the things that you need to do in order to be ready.

Do I really want this?

Why or why not?

Am I ready? Yes/No	
Reasons I am READY	**Reasons I am NOT READY**

WHAT I NEED TO DO TO BE READY

The purpose of this exercise is for you to be able to see what may be holding you back. It is not meant to keep you stuck in your excuses to not move forward. It is meant to help you to see what is needed in order to get to the starting line. I challenge you to try to do these things quickly so you can get started as soon as possible.

You may not be able to do everything on your Need To Do list to be ready. You can however work through or around many of your challenges and get started anyway. Your 'Not Ready' list may be the "safety blanket" that you have been using in order to justify not taking the steps needed to change. You may be scared to face some of your personal issues and that's okay. We're all scared at times but we need to find a way to push through. Often the fear of the unknown or of failure is more paralyzing than just deciding to get going and doing it. Once you start the journey and start feeling lighter (physically and emotionally) you will likely not want to stop and the Not Ready list will not hold the power over you it once did.

The use of a counsellor or support group may also be an option to help you get closer to the core of what is holding you back and preventing you from being ready and getting started. Often we begin to see that it's not what someone did or said to us that keeps us stuck but how we use what others have done and said as a reason for not making changes. You may begin to see that it's YOU holding you back and not what others have said or done to you. No matter what you have experienced in your life, you need to take the steps to change - no one else will do it for you.

If you've decided that you're ready then let's get started as there is lots to do to get ready for your journey to successful weight loss.

Chapter 2

Assembling Your Support Team

I believe that one of the best ways to be successful in your weight loss journey is not to do it alone. It's ultimately up to you to do the work but by having a support system behind you, you will increase the chances that the changes you make will be long lasting, especially through the tough times.

I suggest that you first enlist family, friends and co-workers who have your best interests at heart. They need to be your cheerleaders and be the ones you can talk to when you're stuck or need support. Choose these people carefully as some of them may have their own issues or agendas that could impact your success. If you are able to see a counsellor then I highly recommend it. Often our weight issues are rooted in events from our childhood and past. By reviewing these times, you will likely gain a greater understanding of your relationship with food, exercise and other people. If you can't afford a counsellor, you may want to explore therapists through your work benefits. Also, there may be volunteer counselling or support groups in your community, including online groups.

There is so much conflicting and confusing information out there regarding diet and exercise. Many experts say, eat less, exercise more, drink water, eat less carbs, eat more carbs, eat low fat foods, eat lots of protein, do more cardio, do yoga etc. There is an endless amount of advice, diets and exercise programs out there. Finding the right one for you will take some work on your part. I was able to connect with a dietician through my work benefits. She was very helpful in guiding me towards a healthy, safe and balanced diet. She also was someone who encouraged me to keep going to reach my weight loss and other goals. Some hospitals, health plans and clinics also have dieticians or nutritionists that you may be able to access.

In regards to exercise, if you're able to connect with a personal trainer to guide you at the gym or introduce you to exercising in the community, this is likely your best bet. If you want to start with smaller steps, then walking, riding, or swimming on your own may be where you want to start. Walking groups, pool aerobics, aerobic classes etc. may also be some options. Remember to start at your ability level and where you feel comfortable but make sure it challenges you.

There is also information online about diet and exercise but be careful about what sites you explore and ensure they are reputable and have good reviews by people respected in their field. The more information and support you have, the more powerful and successful you are likely to be. I continue to educate myself about diet and exercise online, in books, magazines, and by asking those I mentioned above. Don't stop your learning as more and better information is constantly coming out.

Chapter 3

Preparing for your Emotional Journey - Writing Your Story

As I prepared to go on my weight loss journey I began realizing that the emotional piece connected to my food addiction needed to be addressed. I began to see that if I did not get to the core of why I was losing and gaining weight year after year, the chances were high that I would continue to yo-yo. I knew how to diet and exercise since I had lost large amounts of weight before. But I didn't know why I continued to gain the weight back. I began to realize the power that I was giving to my emotions and thoughts. They had a hold over me and I needed to get a better understanding of how they were connected to my food addiction.

To gain a better understanding regarding my emotional eating I decided to look back through my life. Often food issues are deeply rooted in experiences from our childhood. I needed to be careful not to use the experiences I had as a child or as an adult as an excuse to continue overeating but rather to help identify old patterns and behaviors. Often, we feel powerless over our past which impacts our present and our future. For me, as long as I could blame those in my past that hurt me I had an excuse to overeat and not take action. I paid for this by remaining obese and unhappy for many years. It wasn't until I took control, stopped blaming and made different choices that I was able to change.

I decided to review my life story with my counsellor first and then write it out fully. I began to see the themes and triggers that influenced my relationship with food. I wrote about times I ate my feelings away and felt numb as well as the times where I chose not to overeat but truly feel my feelings.

The process of writing out my story was powerful and cathartic. It brought up a lot of old feelings I had buried with food and helped me see that I often chose food over experiencing a sad feeling. I began seeing themes and behaviors connected to a difficult experience and overeating. I also saw how I used food to celebrate happy times and how eating became a habit. Food was also a way of being connected during times with family and friends.

Below, you will find a space to write out your own story. Within this story I challenge you to write about the good and bad times as well as what role food played. Here are some questions to ponder:

- Was food scarce?

- Abundant?

- A reward?

- A coping mechanism?

- A habit?

…Or all of the above?

- Did food help you cope with a particular situation or event?

- Did other people in your life have a weight issue?

- Did food become something you enjoyed but it then became a habit that was out of control?

- Can you remember when food began to be more than just nourishment? How did you feel and what did you do?

- Were you scared of your own potential and used food to keep you from being what you dreamed of?

- Did food and weight gain keep people away and protect you in some way?

- Were you made fun of or treated differently for being overweight?

- How did this impact you?

- What about exercise? Was it fun, difficult, or embarrassing?

To give you some ideas on how you may write your story or what it might look like, I have shared mine below. It wasn't easy to write and I had some strong emotional responses to it. You will likely experience numerous emotions in the process of writing your story as well, which is why I recommend talking to a therapist, especially one trained in addiction. Like this book, therapists are there to help you and not to re-traumatize or hold you back.

You will also see how your story can empower you. I challenge you to look at times where things were tough but you made it through anyways; to look at what you did through those times and how you can take the inner strength and resources you gained then and apply it to your food addiction challenge now. First, let's have a look at my story.

My Story

I believe my story around food addiction/emotional eating began even before I was born. My parents had both struggled with their weight as adults. My Mom was thin and healthy when I was born but began gaining weight shortly thereafter. My Dad came from a large family and they liked to eat! I can remember many of them being obese, especially my Uncle Duffy.

My first memory of being the "fat kid" was in 1980. I was 7 and in grade 2. We played a game at school where, while one student left the classroom, the teacher would choose another student who was still in the room to be the "secret student". The child that was out of the room was invited back in, and it was up to the class to provide clues to him/her in order to guess the identity of the secret student.

I was chosen to be the secret student and when my classmate came back into the room, the first clue given to him about me was "he is fat". The student immediately pointed at me. This is one of the first times, other than breaking the plastic ride-on toys as a youngster, that I felt different. I remember my heart sank and I felt tears welling up and a lump in my throat. All the kids laughed. I was devastated.

When I told my parents, they struggled to know what to do for me. The bullying and teasing continued on from there throughout my school years. I did not stand up to the people who bullied me but used food and my sense of humour as a coping strategy; - a deflection. Looking back, I wish I had stood up to the bullying and had the back up from my parents that I needed. Instead, I became the funny, happy kid on the outside but I was often a sad, hurting child on the inside.

I did not tell anyone until I was older about the relentless bullying I endured most days. Not all days were bad and the bullying was more emotional than physical. I was teased for slurring my words and for having a large chest. Clothes didn't fit me well and having a "plumber's bum" at 8 wasn't easy. I was size "husky" and to this day, the word husky bothers me. By today's standards, I wasn't that big. But in the 1980's, I was.

I discovered by grade 5 that I was funny and quick-witted. I used sarcasm as my weapon to strike back at the bullies. I made others laugh about something the bully did so that, if the bully came after me, he looked worse. Now, looking back, I recognize that I was sometimes the bully and I could have responded in a better way.

As a teenager I, much like all the other boys, started liking girls. My friends were getting dates while I always stayed in the "friend-zone." I tried to be what I thought the girls liked; a nice guy who made you laugh and helped with their problems. I lacked confidence and became more jealous and frustrated as my teen years went on. The teasing, and sometimes physical bullying, continued but not around my core group of guy friends who continue to this day to be my best friends. They helped me get through the rest of school and for that I am forever grateful to them.

I was also lucky to have a couple of their mothers who helped me too. Jane and Fran saw that I needed more support and a confidence boost. Jane often gave me advice and would tell me to smarten up when I needed it. I knew it came from a place of love so I was never upset by her. Fran saw potential in me to be someone amazing. She often told me that I was great and would tell me that she was proud of me. Fran listened to my struggles and empathized with me. She always listened and helped me with what I was going through. I called her my 'other Mom' and I continue to be grateful for her every day she was in my life. Fran sadly passed away in 1998. Before she died she told me I would have a great life, be an amazing success and that Alicia and I would live a long, happy life together.

I started trying to lose weight at age 12 and I joined the weight loss group my mom went to. I would not eat on Sunday or Monday in an effort to lose weight for my weekly, Tuesday meeting and weigh in. My Mom would make goals to be thin by Christmas but would never achieve her goal either. I started to try different diets and by high school I was over 200 pounds and had given up. By grade 12, I was 300 pounds.

As a child and teenager I tried to be a perfectionist. I thought that if I didn't make a mistake then there wouldn't be a reason to make fun of me. I didn't like being vulnerable as it was those times I was often picked on the most. I also found myself in the cycle where the bigger I got the more sad I became. The more sad I became the more I ate which caused me to gain even more weight. I found myself becoming addicted to junk food. I was also becoming resigned to a fate of food addiction and sadness. But I also sensed a fire and fight deep inside of me that I hadn't fully found.

My first big weight loss came after a near death experience. In January of 1992, I was 18 years old and had a bad chest cold and bronchitis that I just could not shake. I had dropped out of college and felt like the world's biggest disappointment. I had won scholarships and was to be a successful businessman. I felt pretty low at 300+ pounds.

On February 11, 1992 after 2 days of not sleeping, I told my Dad that I couldn't breathe. He drove me to the hospital where I spent 3 days in intensive care and 4 more days in the hospital. I was scared out of my mind and nearly died. At one point, doctors were preparing to intubate me if I couldn't breathe on my own. While lying alone in the hospital, I told myself I would never be here like this again and I made my first commitment of many to lose the weight.

After being discharged from the hospital, I joined a gym and walked everywhere. I worked at a gas station and got down to 199 pounds. However, once I reached my goal, I started eating unhealthily and continued to party on weekends. I was back up to my heaviest weight within a couple of years. Looking back now, I didn't have the motivation and tools to keep the weight off for the long-term.

After a long term relationship ended in 1995, I decided to remain single. I decided not to rush back into anything with anyone but instead focus on learning about me. I also decided not to try and "fix" whoever I dated next but find someone who was healthy and happy and enjoyed life. I went back to school in 1996 and met the love of my life, and eventual wife, Alicia. Alicia did not have as big of a weight problem as me but over the years we gained weight together. I lost weight for our wedding in 2000 but she didn't. After our wedding I got more into running but a few months into it I felt a pain in my knee. I tried rehabilitating it but I was impatient and gave up. I felt like a victim to my injury and started overeating again. I regained my weight within a year and continued to struggle with yo-yo dieting. I tried many diets including Atkins, Zone Diet and South Beach Diet but couldn't maintain any weight loss I may have had. My weight gain was impacting both myself and my relationship with Alicia. I did not like myself much and continued to struggle with depression. Also, although Alicia and I loved each other deeply, the connection we had was often impacted by the weight we had on us and between us.

In June of 2001 I was hired as a social worker. Over the next few years, I lost and gained 50 plus pounds a few times. Each time, something would happen (injury, let down, life) and I would fall back into my unhealthy patterns of overeating and seeing myself as a victim.

By November of 2008, I tipped the scale at 405 pounds. I was tired of being so big and although I "had it all" (a son, wife, house, picket fence), I still felt unhappy in many ways. I joined a weight loss group that spoke about the emotional challenges of weight loss and I began to lose some weight. I joined a gym and worked out hard, eventually losing 170 pounds. I was on the cover and poster of *The Biggest Loser* (local) contest at my gym. I spoke to the different groups who were involved in the BL Challenge but I still hadn't fully addressed the emotional reasons for my food addiction.

In September of 2009, after many boxing classes, I began feeling a pain in my right shoulder. It was as significant as my knee injury years earlier and I could barely open a door. I went on to make the same mistake of not having a plan for dealing with setbacks. Instead of finding a different way to exercise and work through my disappointment, I said to myself, 'Here I go again', and let the weight come back on by overeating, this time, taking less than a year to gain it all back.

As in the past, I didn't like running into people who had last seen me thin. I could see them look me up and down, debating whether to say anything. I once again felt sad and depressed. I tried hard not to be sarcastic but the worse I ate, the more negative I became. I believed that the world was out to get me as was the black cloud that I thought followed me around. I was again looking to food to help me avoid feeling my emotions. I was so disappointed and upset but did not address it. I blamed everyone else and still couldn't see that the answers were within me. I was caught back in the vicious cycle of being sad because I was so big and then eating to forget about being sad which in turn caused me to gain more weight and be more upset. I hated the way I felt in clothes and dreaded going to restaurants, or theatres unless I could get a chair with a lifting armrest or find a large enough booth.

I felt like I was in a nightmare that I could not wake up from. I worried that I would never be healthy or fit again and I would be stuck at 400 pounds forever. I sweat, all the time. I tried to hunch over to be smaller. I worried about having health complications from being so big. My confidence once again lacked and I felt stuck with no way out. My wife, Alicia, also gained weight and was obese with me. She got healthy before our boys were born but then gained weight again afterwards. I worried about what kind of dad I would be to my sons. What kind of role model was I? By 2010, our finances had tanked and we were not doing anything about it. We continued to eat out at unhealthy restaurants and we drifted in our relationship. Something needed to change.

I needed a new plan; a long-term intelligent plan. I needed a plan on how to eat, exercise and work through physical or mental injuries. I had lots of years of knowledge on how to eat right and exercise. But I continued to ask myself what was missing and how would I get to my goal? I pondered this daily in December of 2014 and decided to give it one last try. I really wanted it and I was ready.

Your Story.

So, now it's time to write your story. I have provided space in the next few pages but feel free to write in a notebook or journal if you need more room. You need to be brutally honest with yourself – looking at the good, bad and ugly. Don't worry about making your writing perfect. Spelling and grammar are not important. Just get your story down on paper as fully and honestly as you can. After you have finished writing, read it over and look for common themes and patterns in your story regarding food, coping, possible trauma, let down, and the overall role that food and exercise played in your life – including food addiction/overeating. You likely can relate to my story in many ways and have other experiences and themes particular to you. I encourage you to check in with your therapist during or after writing your story, especially if you have experienced any type of abuse, neglect, trauma etc. These feelings are powerful and, I believe, to fully work through our weight issues, we need to address the things in our past that we historically chose food to cope with or forget.

For many of us, taking control and not letting our past dictate what we do is one of the first steps in our healing and path to a healthy lifestyle. It can be scary but it is so worth it. It is time to be brave and begin writing and learning about yourself. Once you are able to pick out some of the moments and experiences that impacted your wellbeing you can begin to heal, think differently and make better choices for yourself. You will begin to learn that you are much stronger than you imagined and you have the inner ability to break the emotional grip that your past may have had on you. I will challenge you to identify patterns around your thoughts and behaviors and replace them with new, healthy thoughts and behaviors.

My story began when I was.......

_____

_____

_____

_____

_____

_____

_____

_____

_____

_____

_____

_____

_____

_____

_____

_____

_____

_____

_____

_____

_____

_____

_____

_____

_____

_____

_____

_____

_____

_____

_____

_____

_____

_____

_____

_____

_____

_____

_____

_____

_____

_____

_____

_____

_____

_____

_____

_____

_____

_____

_____

_____

_____

_____

_____

_____

_____

_____

_____

_____

_____

_____

_____

_____

_____

Chapter 4

Identifying Your Themes and Patterns

If you are reading this chapter you have likely finished writing your story. Great job! I imagine it wasn't easy at times but you may also have learned how empowering it is. For many of us, writing our story can be therapeutic as we relive many different emotions and memories. It is my hope that you have begun to identify how truly strong and resilient you are. You have likely been through some very challenging times in your life and prevailed. Now, it's time you begin believing you can do the same with other future challenges including sustained weight loss and creating a long term healthy lifestyle.

An important aspect of understanding your story is being able to identify the themes and patterns that emerged as you were writing. Let's think about my story for a minute. One of the themes that started when I was young was "you're different and not good enough". Being reminded every day that I was fat and that I slurred my words hurt. It hurt a lot. I coped the best I could as a child but even after the teasing stopped, I picked up where others had left off and was overly critical of myself. I felt I needed to be perfect. I did not like being vulnerable, especially at the risk of being hurt more. I gave too much power to what people said about me and I made it my truth even though most of the time it wasn't. Often the hurtful things people said to me were more about them than about me. They were only words. But for a long time I allowed those words to define and limit me.

My self esteem suffered and I ate more to stuff away feelings. I felt stuck and blamed everyone else for where I was in life. Even as an adult I would talk about my past experiences as if they were happening in the present moment. I described them, not as an empowered adult looking back, but more as the hurt child I was then. I knew I needed to work through and process these experiences and feelings in order to break free of the hold they had on me.

Food became my coping mechanism. I ate to numb-out, and the more I ate, the bigger I got. The bigger I got, the more depressed I felt. The more depressed I was, the more I turned to food. I felt trapped in an endless cycle. Whenever I did lose the weight, I didn't have a long-term plan to look forward to. I would get to a goal weight but didn't have any goals beyond that. I wasn't able to (or perhaps I didn't want to) get to the next level of fitness, health and emotional well being. I didn't understand that a large part of keeping weight off and growing as a person was to continue challenging myself to move towards that next level. I will go into Next Level thinking in future chapters.

Another pattern for me was to give up when I faced obstacles. When I got hurt or sick (and you will likely too), I didn't have a plan to work through or around it but instead fell back into being a victim. "Oh, here we go again", I would think. "Daryl luck", I would call it. I didn't find solutions to these challenges. Instead, I would give up exercise and fall back into overeating. I was disappointed and sad like most people would be. But I also wasn't willing, or able, to push through the challenge I faced. And the weight flew back on. I found myself trapped in another endless cycle.

Sometimes when I was trying to lose weight, I would find a reason to quit. I would be feeling down, tired or someone would say or do something hurtful and I chose it as a reason to give up. This behaviour caused many of my starts and stops with my weight loss journey. It was another cycle that I needed to find a way to get out of.

Another theme that I noticed was that I was giving food too much power over me. It was too big a part of my life for all the wrong reasons. If I was happy, I ate. If I was sad, I ate. If it was put in front of me, or if everyone else was eating, I ate no matter how unhealthy it was or how hungry I felt. I didn't want to be deprived or left out, so I ate. What I didn't realize then was that I was really depriving myself of a life free of the constraints of overeating and the negative thoughts and feelings that come along with it. I was also depriving myself of a greater happiness and connection to the world, to my wife, to our children and to myself. I deprived myself of feeling healthy and positive every day. I was not being authentic. I knew I had a greater calling. A happier life was out there for me but I struggled to come out from behind the barriers (both inner and outer) that I had created.

I was a constant people pleaser, protecting other's feelings often at the expense of my own. I worried about everyone's reactions and didn't trust that, if I was respectful but also truthful to who I was, things would likely work out. I thought I was protecting myself and others when really I wasn't truly being who I am. Food helped me numb out when emotions got to be too much. I was kidding myself though and, deep inside me, I knew it. This is when I knew I had to change. The weight loss was going to make me fitter on the outside and hopefully happier on the inside. But what I discovered was that I had to choose to be happy and enjoy the little moments. When I did this, life opened up to me and opportunities presented themselves. It can for you too but you've got to trust in yourself and the process. You can do it!!

Weight loss is not an easy path and you can expect to have many ups and downs emotionally. This is life and how we choose to take on challenges will determine if we are successful. Everyone faces challenges in life and how we cope sets us apart. I would fall back into a victim mode and numb-out with food. I would say things like, "Why me?" and "This doesn't happen to everyone, especially thin, perfect people". Well, I have discovered that everyone has problems and sometimes the 'perfect life' that I think some people have is actually more challenging, in many ways, than mine. Those people who are truly happy appear to accept that good and bad things happen and they need to work through them. A bad situation or event does not ruin their day but they see it as a part of life and often a chance to learn, grow and become stronger.

I continue to learn that my imperfections are a part of me that people can relate to, especially when I am genuine and real. I am not trying to be someone that I am not and I am learning to be vulnerable. For so many years, I tried to be perfect and not let my guard down in case someone made a mean or embarrassing comment towards me. As I have stated earlier, I now understand that what people say is often more about them and what they're going through than it is about me.

I also realized that unhealthy food was giving me a hangover type of feeling the next day. I felt negative, sick, depressed and lacked energy the following morning after binging. I craved more unhealthy food and it would take me a couple of days to feel positive again.

Looking back at your story, I strongly recommend that you work to identify the themes and patterns in your life. I encourage you to bring these insights to your therapist or counsellor and go deeper into them. Looking at your patterns and themes can be humbling but it can also be a way to see how you have moved through challenges in the past, especially the times where you didn't overeat.

I challenge you to embrace and honour your story, and don't allow it to be the reason for not moving forward on your journey. Avoid the urge to stuff these feelings away, especially with food. The goal is to find a balance of feeling through difficult feelings, gaining insight, and then moving towards your goals. Knowledge is power and it can help you to respond in a healthy way when old feelings/habits/behaviours rear their heads. This will allow you to choose new behaviours and create new habits.

In coming chapters you will be empowered to choose a different path and replace old behaviours with new healthier ones. Begin by starting to think about how you will respond differently to situations without using food. Then, challenge yourself to use these strategies when the opportunity arises in your life.

Now, I would like you to review your story. On the next page, write out your themes/patterns as well as the impact it had on you – good, bad or indifferent. Then come back to the New Behaviour as you read through the book. You may have new behaviours already in your head to write but also be open to creating new ones.

Themes/Patterns/ Behaviours	Impact or effect	Possible New Behaviour
eg. I would fall back into emotional eating after getting physically or emotionally hurt.	I typically gained back the weight I lost plus more. I felt worse about myself and it would take years for me to pull out of it and get back to a healthy weight.	Talk about and feel through my disappointment. Also find new ways of exercising until my injury healed.

Chapter 5

Picking Your Start Date

If you haven't already, it's now time to pick a start date and create some initial goals for your journey to successful weight loss. Once you have chosen a start date it is imperative that you DON'T keep moving the date back. In the past, I would always start on a Monday and then if there was some type of dessert at work or if I had a rough day I would often decide to eat the treat or find one which then would lead me back to old unhealthy eating habits. I would start again on the next Monday hoping that the same thing wouldn't happen again. When I chose to have a large unhealthy treat I believed that I had screwed up the entire week anyway so I might as well go for it and eat whatever I want. I would end up gaining more weight and feeling worse.

I began thinking about how to stop this cycle. What worked for me was to change my "all or nothing" thinking. I would often try to eat flawlessly when I started a diet. It was either I ate perfectly or just went for it with unhealthy choices. I now realize that I don't have to be perfect. Now, I allow myself to emotionally let go of "unhealthy" food choices I have made and get right back on track immediately rather than waiting until Monday to start again. I don't beat myself up or go on a five day food bender. Eventually, you will be able to have a small piece of cake or donut (if you choose to) but then make a healthier choice right after. This is what I often observed healthy people doing and it seems to work. They often go for a walk after eating so they don't gain any weight and still feel good afterwards rather than experiencing the bloated/negative feelings that come with binging.

Remember now that if you have a small piece of dessert or decide not to it's not because you can't but because you have made a choice. You need to take your power of choice back. When I feel I *can't* eat something, I want it more. However, when I *choose* to have it or not, I maintain my power. People may try to pressure you and you need to be kind but firm and thank them for the offer but you're choosing not to have it today. I would often say this then have something healthy while finding a conversation to join. I began to see that I could be at a social function and eat healthy or not at all. I made the function about the people and not the food. I felt empowered, especially after I reflected back about the day.

So, pick your date and stick to it! If you want a "last supper", go for it but do not keep having them. You will likely make some unhealthy choices and this is part of the weight loss journey. It is not a perfect path but staying as close as you can to it will help you to be more successful. Get right back to your healthy eating plan with your next meal. Don't beat yourself up if you had an unhealthy meal or day. Just get back on track right away. You will thank yourself the next day and not feel trapped in the cycle of eating healthy and then binging.

Once you have picked your day, you will likely feel excited and motivated. Know that this excitement will likely lessen over time. The secret will be knowing how to keep motivated, work through challenges and not be discouraged by times of slower progress. Remember, you have the resources and tools within you to do this no matter what gets thrown at you. You will also likely have the support of some family, friends and co-workers. Some may be more supportive than others, so be cautious who you pick in your weight loss support circle. There may be some family/friends who want to keep you where you're at so they feel better while others may be critical or not fully understanding of what you're going through. As I've said, weight loss groups, nutritionists, dieticians, trainers, etc. can often be excellent supports as well.

Chapter 6

Preparing for Challenges

I can almost guarantee you that throughout your weight loss journey you will be faced with challenges that could (if you choose) derail your progress. I thought about this and how I could plan ahead to take on challenges to help ensure that I did not fall into my old way of being (overeating after a disappointment or injury). By being prepared and ready for the challenges I faced, I was able to stay on track.

I want to warn you that some days are going to be tough. You will realize, as I did, that in the long run, getting through those tough days are worth it as they will show you that you can get through anything. You will become physically and emotionally stronger and challenges that threw you off before will have less impact. The key will be to keep moving forward no matter what is thrown at you. Stay disciplined, but also be human and learn from your challenges and mistakes. Making mistakes is part of the fun and process. Resist the urge to put yourself down if you make a mistake. Instead see mistakes as an opportunity to learn and grow. Remember, by working through the tough times you're doing what others only wish they were doing. Each time you do this you take another step closer to your goal.

Another mistake I made was that I was not prepared for an injury or illness. In the past I had used both of these as an excuse to give up. As you lose weight, you will likely challenge yourself physically with new exercises and injuries may happen. You may also get a flu or cold that will slow down your progress. By seeing that injury and illness can often be worked around until you're well, you will be less likely to give up or revert to old behaviours. Professional athletes would not have careers if they let an injury stop them every time they got hurt.

I refused to be complacent and slide back into my old habits. I had moments that I did but I only stayed there for a short period of time. I started thinking to myself, "What would happen if I continued to eat junk?" I realized, and became really worried, that I would fall back into my old eating habits and the weight would come back. This fear became greater than my fear of not having junk food. I realized junk food was bringing me down and I would no longer let this happen. I took a stand against eating unhealthy food, as it only brings a quick high and resulted in a longer term feeling of sadness and being stuck.

Another change in my mindset that helped me prepare for my weight loss journey and the challenges that came along with it was deciding to take care of me. Many people who struggle with their weight are selfless caregivers that give, give, give and forget that they need to take care of themselves first in order to best serve others. Being of service to people is a very rewarding way of life but it shouldn't be at the expense of your own well being. You deserve to be happy and get the most out of life as much as anyone else. Being a victim or martyr may give you some pay off but it eventually breeds resentment and then nobody is happy. Don't think that by putting yourself first and saying 'no' to people is selfish. You must no longer abandon yourself but instead, make yourself and your needs the first priority. Many of us have taken care of others at the expense of our own well-being. I have learned that by caring for myself first (including my health and emotional well being), I am way more effective in helping others and have improved in almost all other areas of my life. The challenges I face now don't feel so daunting as I see them as a learning opportunity and not as something that I will allow to bring me down.

Chapter 7

Specific Goal Setting

I can't emphasize enough how important goal setting is. What worked for me was to have both small goals and larger ones. The realization that goal setting was a lifelong process, and not just something I did until I reached my goal weight, was incredibly helpful. It is very important that the goals you make are specific with measurable results. Having a goal date to achieve your goals by also helps you be accountable to yourself and those you share with. Goals can be adjusted for unforeseen circumstances but you need something really specific to aim for. General goals are good but sometimes more difficult to measure.

It is important to set goals that are both challenging yet achievable for you. Saying that I wanted to lose 100 pounds in 6 months felt too big for me. But chunking it up into smaller goals (10-15 pounds a month) felt less overwhelming and I celebrated each small goal that I met. For example, you may want to make a goal of losing 8-10 pounds in a month or that you want to be down 2 dress sizes. Your goals don't all have to be weight related; to stop drinking pop, lower your blood pressure or be off your diabetes medication etc. can also be goals you strive for.

Another key piece to goal setting is to make sure that you continually review your goals and make any shifts necessary and then create new goals. I continue to create new and bigger goals today so I never feel stagnant or the desire to fall backwards. New goals keep things fresh and exciting. When you do something you had previously only dreamed about you will likely get hooked and go on to the next exciting challenge. Often, we sell ourselves short. But once we realize there is another life out there and it's ours for the taking at any age, the world will open up to thousands of possibilities. I'm not just saying this. I have been in a dark place before. But now I can say I enjoy living a life full of possibilities. Trust in the process you are in and you too will see things differently.

As I prepared for my weight loss journey, I sat down and asked myself "What do I want to achieve?" The big mistake I had made before (and hope you can avoid) was having a single goal, for example, being at a certain weight or be thin for a wedding. When you only have one big goal, the little challenges can seem overwhelming and it's easy to fall back into victim mode and put the weight back on.

What I have learned is that goals need to be fluid and never ending. Now, if I reach one goal or get near it, I'm already and automatically thinking of the next goal. My overall goal was to become healthy and stay healthy; not just until I reached my goal weight or my nephew's wedding day, but to continue building on and learning about nutrition, physical health and improving my emotional well-being. I now understand that by always thinking of new goals and being hungry (no, not that kind of hunger... but a drive to get to the next level) I could achieve my goals and dreams.

I am now at a point in my journey where I look ahead to achieving goals that I never thought possible; things like writing this book and doing sporting events. You will see that your outlook on life, energy and overall well being will improve. You might ask yourself why you didn't do this before. But don't beat yourself up about it. You needed to go through whatever it was for a reason and it helped to create who you are today. Positive and not so positive experiences all have lessons to teach us. The key is not only how we interpret our experiences and learn from them, but it's also having gratitude for all we have been through. Putting your goals and desires out there in writing and then acting upon them is the first step to making things happen (including weight loss). It's not just waiting until you've got things figured out in your head. It's also about acting on your goals right in this moment. It may sound hokey, but when I say something is going to happen and then start taking the steps towards it, things happen and I realize how powerful I really am. You are powerful too!

Meeting both smaller and larger goals will give you an amazing sense of accomplishment. Once you begin reaching one goal, write down a new one. Don't stop reaching for that next level in diet, exercise and emotional wellbeing. Also, writing down a goal rather than having it just in your head helps in cementing the commitment you made. It's there for you to review and share with others if you wish.

When I look back at what I set out to achieve, I begin to see I often went farther than many of the goals I created. I started feeling unstoppable. Having a written record to review will remind you just how far you have come, especially on those days when you may be feeling down. Writing down goals is also like a contract with yourself. If you break this contract you're really only letting yourself down. Crossing off a written goal also gives you a sense of pride and a visual of what you're capable of doing and where you want to go.

When I got close to my goal weight I saw that I had potential to do even bigger things like endurance races, Tough Mudder runs, sports, writing a book, job promotion, whatever I put my mind to. Eating healthy and exercising kept my brain and emotions positive and I was less likely to listen to the other voice in my head telling me I couldn't do it. Whatever your goal is, once you get there, you will realize that there are even bigger goals and dreams at your fingertips waiting for you to take action. Saying your goals out loud with positive affirmations like "I'm powerful" or "I'm unstoppable" will also help you create the results you desire.

I now encourage you to start writing out your own plan and goals (see example and place to start creating goals on page 44). Feel free to use some of my ideas and create some of your own goals that will help set you up to be successful. Also, use a notebook or My Fit Pal (online food journal) to keep track of all the pieces of your journey: your food journal, your exercise schedule and your emotions connected to food. At the front of your book, you may want to include your initial weight and inches (waist, neck, arms legs, etc.) as well as your goals – long term and short term.

Overall First Goal: eg. lose 150 pounds

Smaller Goal 1: eg. start riding my exercise bike 25 minutes a day

Goal 2: eg. stop eating processed foods full of sugar and flour

Goal 3: eg. limit eating dessert to once a week

Next Level – New goals.

Goal 1. eg. join a gym and go 3 times minimum a week.

Goal 2. eg. do a 5 KM walk run with a group of friends

Overall First Goal:

Smaller Goal 1:

Goal 2:

Goal 3:

Overall Second Goal:

Goal 1:

Goal 2:

Goal 3:

Chapter 8

Preparing for DAY 1

In preparing for day 1, it is important to set yourself up for success by doing some planning and organizing. It should be noted that any change in diet and exercise should be discussed with a doctor or other health professional before starting. If you have any type of health issues, discuss them further with a health professional to ensure your medical safety. For those with or without medical issues, you may want to get some routine tests done as a baseline (such as resting heart rate, blood pressure, blood sugar, cholesterol, etc.). You could get these done again in six months and/or a year to also track your progress. I did this when I was down 80 pounds and my results were amazing. My results also gave me a boost to continue to improve and learn more about health.

I purchased a quality bathroom scale. I suggest you do the same. It is a good idea to weigh yourself at the beginning so that you know your starting point. Also, take some basic size measurements such as your neck, chest, waist, thighs etc. As time goes on, your weight loss will likely slow a bit, so tracking inches lost and how you feel in your clothes will help you see and track progress other than what the scale says. You will likely gain muscle too. So if you're losing inches but the weight stays the same for a while don't panic. However, if your weight stays the same or goes up and you're not losing inches, it's time to reevaluate what you're eating and the kinds of exercise you are doing. I could do three workouts in a day but if my eating was not healthy I still gained weight. I could lose weight without exercising but it was slower and I did not feel as good if I didn't include exercise. I used the scale as a tool and modified how I used it to fit my needs.

Choosing how often you weigh yourself will be up to you. The scale is a tool of measurement and should NOT be used as a tool to decide if you are happy or worthy. The scale does not decide if you are having a good day or not. I tracked my food and calories every day by writing it down in my food journal or in My Fit Pal. I also weighed myself every day too. I knew my weight would not go down every day and that I would plateau or even go up on occasion. I used the scale to help me see if what I was eating and the exercise that I was doing was helping over time. The scale would help me see patterns and if I needed to make adjustments to what I was eating and how much I exercised. The scale, combined with how my clothes fit me and measurements I had taken, helped me see where I was at.

Please be cautious and back off the scale if you find you are getting obsessive about it or if it is impacting your moods! As I mentioned before, if your weight stays the same and your clothes are tight, then have another look at what you are eating and how much you are exercising. If you would rather weigh yourself once a week, that works just as well. Another scale tip is to only weigh once a day or week and weigh yourself at the same time each day/week. You typically will weigh less in the morning.

Eating Plan

One of the first things I did before my start date was to clear my cupboards, pantry, fridge, freezer and secret hiding spots (you know you have them) of any kind of junk food. My wife and I bought fruits, vegetables, yogurt (plain, not low-fat), chicken, fish, tofu, turkey, eggs, salad mix of different leafy vegetables, oatmeal and cheese.

I began reading articles on health and health foods. I also watched Youtube and Netflix documentaries on food (see a list of my favourites in the resource section at the end of the book). I was surprised by how much information there was. I also read about the benefits of drinking lemon water as well as cinnamon and local honey in warm water. I began drinking these first thing in the morning to help flush my system. I am not a big alcohol drinker and never smoked cigarettes but I loved soda pop. I thought Coke Zero™ was a healthier choice than the regular Coke™ but after researching artificial sweeteners, I began to understand that they were actually worse than the sugar in regular soda. I knew I had to stop drinking it, so I decided to slowly wean myself off of it, being completely pop-free by the end of January 2015. To my surprise pop actually started tasting like chemicals and not matching up with the benefits of the natural healthy choices I was making.

My research also led me to limit my refined sugar, processed food and flour intake. I looked to healthy carbs and starches and avoided some carbohydrates. I began jokingly saying at work, "carbs are the devil" when there were cookies and cake in the lunchroom. It should be noted that carbs like fruits, veggies and some whole grains in moderation are not the devil. Many carbs are actually healthy and needed in order to help give you brain power.

You may also want to start looking at calorie intake. Choosing healthy foods including lots of raw fruits and vegetables will fill you up. Remember to also eat enough so that you do not starve your body. When you starve yourself, your body reacts to the lack of fuel and tells itself that there is a famine, essentially hanging on to the fat for the upcoming lack of food. I recommend that you consult your doctor or a dietician or nutritionist regarding diet, caloric intake etc. to ensure your overall health needs are met.

I feared being deprived of the junk food I enjoyed. I knew I had to let go of the all or nothing mentality and it seemed that most people went off healthy eating plans when they felt deprived. So, I decided I would plan ahead and give myself one "treat" not "cheat" day. I learned that having something I enjoyed, like popcorn, was not a bad thing unless it became a binge day. I did not like the term "cheat day" as it had the connotation of being negative/bad. I would choose my treat day around social events so I could have what I wanted and not feel deprived (eg, being the only one eating lettuce and skipping the nachos). I wasn't ready to make the shift yet to being okay with eating from the veggie tray and not having a treat with everyone else.

When we are deprived, we often want more of what we are not allowed to have. I began to realize that I needed to see this differently and have a new relationship with all food. This would be a process and I wouldn't have it all figured out in the first day. I decided at the beginning of my journey that I would only have one treat day a week and if I really wanted a piece of birthday cake in the middle of the week, it would be a small piece.

As I mentioned before, I watched how people who are healthy ate and took on some of their characteristics. I saw that they would have a small piece of cake but then go back to veggies and go for a walk in the afternoon. The people who are healthy never said, "Oh, I wrecked it now", and start eating everything. They could enjoy a treat but then maintain healthy eating and exercising right after the small piece of cake. I decided to try this strategy as well.

Keeping a Food Journal:

To help me get a better picture of what I ate, how I felt and how it impacted me, I decided to start journaling my food every day. I could see that sometimes, if I had a bad day or felt deprived, I would eat unhealthy foods. Once I had a better understanding and awareness of my eating habits and how they were connected to my food, I began challenging myself to actually feel my feelings rather than numbing out with junk food. I also made healthy choices during these times and learned that I actually felt better when I ate well even if I was experiencing difficult emotions. I also discovered that, if I was able to eat healthily and feel full, my craving for unhealthy food and sad/frustrated feelings went away. Sometimes it was just about getting through the tough times and learning that they really weren't as bad as I thought. Junk food wasn't really helping me but actually bringing me further down. Maybe I had a quick food high but like other drugs the high went away fast and I would be constantly trying to get high again. I discovered a new high consisting of power foods and exercise and learned that these were what my body and mind really craved not cake or ice cream as I once thought.

Food Journal Example

Date: For the week of _____.

Weight:

Measurements: Chest Waist Biceps Hips Upper leg Calves etc.

Day:

Breakfast (include; mood/feelings/situation):

Snack (mood/feelings/situation):

Lunch (mood/feelings/situation):

Snack (mood/feelings/situation):

Supper (mood/feelings/situation):

Liquids:

Exercise:

Notes:

So, before Day 1 comes, start creating a diet plan and develop some strategies that will support regular, healthy nutrition. Some strategies may be clearing your home of junk food, buying foods recommended by your doctor, nutritionist and/or dietician. Again, the help of a professional can get you on the right track and help set up an eating plan that feels right for you - one where you don't feel deprived and that you believe will be sustainable over the long-term. There are also many books on healthy eating and information on the internet. Be cautious of anything too drastic and check the sources. I did limit some of my carb intake but this was mostly with processed sugars and flour. I still ate fruits, vegetables and created my own ancient grain cereal. Remember that this is not just a diet that you will be on until you reach your goal weight. This is a lifestyle change. So, make sure that it is something you can enjoy but also gives the best nutritional bang for your buck. Serving sizes and exactly what you eat will also depend on your activity level, age, gender and any health needs you may have. I'm cautious to tell you exactly what to eat here as everyone is different. For me, I did my own research and began incorporating superfoods into my eating plan. I drank plenty of water and avoided eating after 8 PM. I will share more regarding my health changes as I take you through my 12 month transformation.

You also need to start considering the kinds of exercise that you want to start doing. This is important to help ensure that you are both challenged by the exercise you're doing and gaining benefits without overdoing it or burning out.

Exercise Plan

Developing my new exercise plan was next. I enjoy watching *The Biggest Loser* and *Extreme Make Over Weight Loss Edition* but what I found was that the contestants were made to start exercising too intensely for their fitness level, their size and their athletic ability. If you have a personal trainer pushing you each day and a doctor monitoring your health, then this may be ok. But if you're doing this on your own or with limited support, then you need to do what works for you to be successful. I recommend a personal trainer or health coach to help you get started on an exercise plan that meets your needs.

I started with a goal to exercise 4-5 times per week. I would do exercises that I liked and at a pace that challenged me but did not overwhelm me or burn me out. I would naturally and steadily increase my exercise level and celebrate my successes. I would also find people to teach, motivate and cheer me along to help me stay focused and excited.

Whether you are a former professional athlete, Olympian, high school or college star, or have never really exercised, everyone can exercise and everyone can become athletic. Yes, this is true and you will eventually start to see yourself as an athlete. With a good program, tailored for you, you will start to challenge yourself to go to the next fitness level. The trick is to not let yourself stay stagnant. If your routine gets easy, then change it up and increase the resistance level. This may mean going with heavier weights, different exercises, or, in regards to cardio, increasing your duration and intensity.

I suggest you start by picking a low impact exercise like walking, (treadmill or outdoors), stationary bike riding or elliptical training. For me at nearly 400 pounds I couldn't go running the first day as it would have been too hard on my joints and I would have likely given up or stopped altogether. Depending on your age, weight and size, you may want to start with 10-20 minutes. Like your food plan, everyone is different so I don't want to give you exact exercises to do. I would rather have you do exercises that you like already or have a fitness expert show you a plan. If personal trainers are not in your budget, then things like riding your bike, going for challenging walks or hikes or swimming may be some options. There are often different types of aerobic classes that are affordable as well. Just get your heart rate up and get moving. For me the automatic interval setting on the cardio machines at the gym worked well when I first started. I set the resistance hard for one minute and then low resistance the next minute. The intervals brought my heart rate up and down, causing me to burn more calories. I did not start with an exceptionally high pace. Nor did I set the bar too low. I felt good afterwards but not exhausted. I would try and walk and stretch daily. As my endurance started to improve, I would exercise harder. If the intensity of your workout is too much, go slower for longer. You will still burn calories and likely not be as easily discouraged. Remember to consult with your doctor or health professional before starting a new exercise plan. Having fun and staying motivated is also highly recommended.

I like music that pumps me up with a good beat for exercising. I have found good music on *YouTube*. I also looked for motivational speakers combined with my music. I listened to many motivational speakers while I rode my stationary bike. I found that my way of thinking started to change. Many of the speakers spoke about hard work, integrity, perseverance, overcoming adversity and doing the work that people on the couch were wishing they could do. By staying consistent with healthy eating and exercise you will make this shift from the couch to whatever you decide you want to do. I can't say enough about how healthy eating and regular exercise will change your confidence and overall outlook on life. For me, unhealthy food kept me down and depressed while healthier foods and exercise helped me become powerful. It takes work and discipline but as I keep saying, it's so worth it!

There will be days where you won't feel like exercising. We all have these days. What I found was that when I pushed myself to go anyways I was grateful and felt better for it, often within minutes of starting. There will be days where you need to rest and if you're worn out I suggest you listen to your body and take a break. However, on the days you just feel lazy, you need to push yourself. I stuck to my schedule and honoured my commitment to exercise which helped me move towards my goals. I also felt better equipped to take on the challenges the day presented to me. My attitude and confidence were often much higher than if I did nothing.

The Gym

At nearly 400 pounds, the gym can be intimidating place both from a mental and social perspective. I felt self-conscious especially around those who were already strong and fit. I decided to go anyway and try not to worry about everyone else but do what I needed for me. Then one afternoon, in the middle of my workout, a strong, muscular guy who I had seen many times before came up to me. He gave me some words of encouragement and noticed that I was losing weight. I made some kind of self-deprecating remark about my size and he responded by saying that he had more respect for people coming to the gym, whatever size they were, than if he saw them going into a fast food restaurant. This helped me worry less about what others thought. I started being a little more outgoing in the gym and others also started encouraging me and noticing the changes I was making.

You can tailor your workout to what works for you. If you're a novice in the gym, then have a trainer set up a program for you and show you proper technique. I have learned that how much you lift is not nearly as important as proper technique/form and consistency. I also learned that doing different exercises would keep my body guessing and needing to use different parts of each muscle. Your body will adjust to your routine so keep changing it up so your body is always guessing and needing to repair itself (this is where muscles grow and become stronger). This also goes for doing different types of cardio.

You need to be aware that exercise may not be comfortable at first, especially if you have more than 50 pounds to lose. Sometimes it sucks and this is where people will give up. The ability to push through and stay consistent will get you the results you desire. It takes time and each workout will get you another step closer to your goal. Like healthy eating, the more consistent you are, the better the results. Also, if you miss a workout don't give up, just get back the next day rather than waiting to start again on Monday. You will feel better for it.

Eventually as you get closer to your goal weight, you will begin looking for new and exciting challenges like runs, hikes, marathons, bike races, Tough Mudders, Crossfit classes, Foam Runs, sport teams, running clubs, boot camps, just to name a few. There are many, many exciting activities out there that you can be a part of and should be a part of. Don't limit yourself; dream big, plan and go for it!

I like to walk, hike, and now run. I listen to my body and don't push it if I feel a twinge somewhere or I feel overly tired. I suggest that if you want to run you take a running course and are at a weight that will not put too much stress on your joints.

If the gym is not for you that's 100% okay. It's not <u>where</u> you work out but more that you <u>do</u> work out. The gym is one of many places you can go to get exercise. Lifting weights has shown in many studies I have read to be beneficial to keeping bones strong and avoiding decay of muscles. You can buy weights or machines to use at home too. It's ultimately up to you.

Emotional and Psychological Preparation

An old Cherokee is teaching his grandson about life. "A fight is going on inside me," he said to the boy.

"It's a terrible fight and it is between two wolves. One is evil - he is anger, envy, sorrow, regret, greed, arrogance, self-pity, guilt, resentment, inferiority, likes, false pride, superiority, and ego." He continued, "The other is good - he is joy, peace, love, hope, serenity, humility, kindness, benevolence, empathy, generosity, truth, compassion, and faith. The same fight is going on inside you - and inside every other person, too."

The grandson thought about it for a minute and then asked his grandfather, "Which wolf will win?"

The old Cherokee simply replied, "The one you feed."

As I mentioned earlier, in preparation for my weight loss journey I also began addressing the emotional and psychological challenges that had been impacting my ability to lose and keep weight off. I started counselling even before my start date in order to get the underlying reasons why I was addicted to food. I addressed my all or nothing thinking and tendency to compare myself to thin people who I labeled as "perfect". I watched a Ted Talk featuring Brene Brown who stated that, "People who were whole hearted embraced vulnerability and they believed what made them vulnerable made them beautiful." My therapist and I worked on the difference between so-called "perfect" people and real people. She asked me who I liked better and I said "real" people. I explained that people appeared to be more attracted to me when I was genuine rather than who I thought they wanted me to be. I began to see that being vulnerable (making mistakes, showing emotion) wasn't so scary but were often times where I felt the most alive.

As I stated before, writing my story and looking at themes and patterns connected to my food addiction was sometimes emotionally painful. It brought back old memories that weren't easy for me but I also gained strength from it as I began seeing the strength I possessed to take on other challenges in my life. I began seeing that I could let my past memories beat me or I could allow them to teach me. I also started seeing that those who were hurtful to me were also in pain, sometimes more. And that what they did or said to me was more about what was going on for them than me. Their words were not my truth. I realized that for many years I let what they said define me and hold me back but I was not going to do this any longer. I knew who I was on the inside and now, more than ever, I needed to express it. I had used food for too long to suppress all my emotions and now

I would be going on a journey to wellness. The more I learned about myself, the more I felt prepared for what was ahead. By changing my thinking about myself and the world I began to see that food wasn't trapping me but my choices were. I did not need to be at the mercy of my emotions but instead I could choose how I felt and responded to my past, present and future.

I knew that there were days ahead that would challenge me to my limits. I was about to go through a transformation and I had to trust that on the other side was the life I dreamed of and deserved. I no longer was going to give myself the option of eating my feelings but instead feeling them. I was, in a sense, giving up my safety blanket and this was scary but exciting at the same time. I had had enough of being morbidly obese and I knew that if I were to break free I had to be brave and not use food to cope. All my research, training and counselling had prepared me for the path I was about to take. I had to trust the process and take it day by day. My thoughts about myself were changing as were my thinking around diet and exercise. I was going into this, not on a whim, but with support and a plan. I had learned that good planning often produces good results. I had more confidence in what was possible in the coming months because I had prepared for it and was going to do it methodically and with intention. I had a renewed sense of energy and I had the support and mindset needed to be triumphant.

Going in with a positive mindset definitely helped me but did not prepare me for everything. I understood that, like any journey, going in unprepared would likely end up in disappointment including gaining the weight back. The stubborn side of me said that this wasn't going to happen again and I would draw strength from my inner resources. It was time to be courageous and I was ready.

I continued to learn about myself and challenge myself to feel through difficult times. I did not let setbacks set me back but instead found ways around them. I did not give up or give in and it was very tough as the little voice on my shoulder tried to pressure me to eat junk food. I believed that chocolate and pastries would make me feel better when all they did was give me a small sugar high. I found that I was right back to feeling down in no time. When I made the choice to commit to my healthy eating plan I wouldn't listen to the negative voice but instead chose to eat healthy and exercise. I listened to the other voice that said to make the choices that will best serve me. I believe everyone has this inner voice but often we let the negative voice win. This time I wasn't going to let my negative self talk be my master and somewhere inside me I knew this for sure.

You too need to find and listen to your positive voice; the voice that encourages you to make healthy choices and fight through desires to overeat. At one time the negative voice served a purpose and met a need. However, as you eat healthy and find effective ways to cope, you will discover that the negative voice no longer serves you and is actually bringing you down. Sometimes when you're tired or busy it's hard to listen to the positive voice and this is when you need to slow yourself down and listen to what your body and mind are screaming at you to do.

I challenge you to start changing the way you see things in preparation for your journey. Prepare for battle not only on the outside with attaining your supports and adjusting your environment but also prepare yourself on the inside too. As I have learned, you can do everything on the outside to be ready but until you take control of your emotions, the chances of returning to your old unhealthy ways is almost certain.

In the next chapters, you will read what I did to successfully lose 155 pounds. This can be your path too. I hope that, by reading further about what I did, you will be prepared and be successful in your weight loss journey. So, let's go....

Chapter 9

Getting Started

You are probably feeling really excited about the journey you are about to undertake. You may also feel some fear around making some pretty big changes. Like the negative inner voice, fear of the future does not serve much purpose. Try not to let your fear impact you, but rather focus your energy on your next steps. Now it's time to choose your start date and commit to not changing it. For me, I chose January 1, 2015. You don't need to wait until January 1st or some other date that seems significant. Just get started as soon as you can. Also, remember that this exciting feeling will fade a little but does come back. Not many people can maintain the excitement from when they begin. I found as I lost the weight and began feeling better, the excitement came back. It's what people do in the in between times that separates the people who achieve their goals from those who don't.

So, before you officially start, let's ensure that you have written out why you're ready to do this as well as your story about you and food. You have picked out the themes/behaviours regarding emotional overeating. You have thought about and talked to either a trusted friend or counsellor about your past behaviours and emotions with food. You have set up an eating and exercise plan, including a food journal or have My Fit Pal set up. You have consulted your doctor and you have also spoken with a nutritionist or dietician. You have also consulted a personal trainer or done research on exercise including easily available activities that you enjoy. Your support circle is ready to support you. You have created and committed to your long and short term goals with a plan to create new ones as you complete initial goals. You have prepared yourself emotionally for the journey you're about to go on. You also have some ideas around what you're going to do differently when you have a craving, a bad day or want to give up. Finally, you have done your measurements, weighed yourself and reviewed your checklist one last time.

Remember that, if you need to, you can go back to the beginning of the book and start doing the steps again. This is key if you find yourself falling back into old habits of overeating or binge eating. There is no judgement, as this is a tough journey and sometimes it takes some setbacks to get where we want to go.

My hope is that as you read my experience you will be able to relate, gain strategies and learn what to expect in the coming months. I also hope to inspire you to keep moving ahead. So take a deep breath and let's get started. It's likely going to be one of the most challenging, but also one of the most rewarding, things you ever do.

Week 1

Good morning and welcome to Week 1. Week one, especially day one, is often very exciting. You're likely filled with lots of anticipation about where your journey is going to take you. If you have followed all the steps, you're likely set up and are ready to change your life. Remember to eat enough and to start your exercise activity. Expect that this week you will probably drop a good amount of weight. Also expect that in week two that you will drop a lot less. Often our bodies will lose water the first week and then try to level itself out. This is natural and typical so don't get discouraged. Your cravings are likely to start after a day or two as well, so incorporating your new strategies and supports is vital to maintain your new behaviours. It is likely that you may go to work or for a visit at a friend's place and a treat may be offered to you. This happened to me on day two. I was polite to the person offering me a snack but used my power of choice to say no thank you. It will be tough at first to say no and not want to offend the person offering, but if they are truly a friend they will understand. I would tell people that I

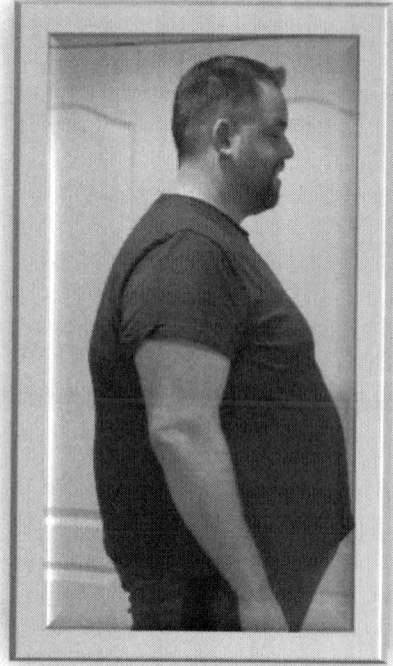

started a new healthy eating program and that I was limiting my intake of sugars and processed food. People would sometimes ask if there was anything else I might like and I would ask about veggies or fruit or just a glass of water.

As I have said, if you're more than 50 pounds overweight, exercise is likely going to be tough. Pick an activity that you enjoy and that challenges you but doesn't burn you out. Too many times people want to run a marathon right away but this takes time to build up to. Be patient. The more consistent you are with healthy eating and exercising the faster you will get to your physical and emotional goals. I found that I was sore after exercising as I was quite overweight and out of shape but I also pushed myself to stay at it and it did not take long to get results. As I saw results, I was inspired to push ahead for more.

There is some debate about whether a treat day is a wise thing to do. I say it depends on who you are and how a treat day impacts you. I found for myself that having a treat day and matching it up with a social event helped me. I still got to enjoy a treat but I chose what it was and how much of it I ate. However, at the beginning, I think I still ate too much. After my first treat day I gained 4 pounds of the seven I had lost that week. This impacted my mood, motivation and overall outlook so I had to be careful that I didn't fall back into old habits or making unhealthy choices. After a treat day or treat meal I made a decision that I would eat healthily the next day even if I had the urge to eat junk. I found that the weight I gained came off fairly fast and that I felt better quicker if I started eating well right away. I also took note of how an unhealthy eating day impacted me and knew that I would likely need to adjust what a treat day looked like as the weeks went on.

My first week went well and I already felt a sense of pride and accomplishment. I also saw that by being prepared, putting everything together that I knew about weight loss and then setting it into action, I had the potential to have long term success in my journey. I still was a little fearful of falling back into emotional overeating but something told me to just keep doing what I needed to do each day and that I would get there.

When I weighed myself after the first week, I had lost 7 pounds and felt great. I liked to weigh myself everyday as a guide to see if I had to make any adjustments to my diet and activity level. Be cautious not to use the scale as a measure of your worthiness. See Chapter 8 for more information on scale use.

If you followed the plan closely, you are likely down 4 - 8 pounds at the end of week 1. Know that this likely will not happen every week, especially in week 2. Week 1 is often a big loss as your system doesn't know what hit it and responds very favourably. If you haven't lost any weight, review your diet and exercise journal. Was your treat meal too much? Did you exercise? Did you exercise enough? Did you eat too many processed foods or not enough food? Talk to a dietician, nutritionist or a personal trainer for more ideas to adjust your diet and exercise program.

Week 2

As I mentioned before, be prepared for your week 2 weight loss to be less than week 1. This is normal. Be happy with any loss this week and stay on track. Your body is likely adjusting to the change and holding onto fat, muscle, water etc. until it knows it's not experiencing a famine. By staying active and eating right, your body will grow and repair to be a healthier you. This is not a sprint but a process that takes time. I suggest at least 5 days a week for some form of exercise.

I also got into watching food documentaries on Netflix about health. Some of these videos included "Forks Over Knives", "Fat, Sick, & Nearly Dead", and "Food Matters." As I watched the movies, I started picking out common themes around eating superfoods and the benefits they have for your body and mind. I started adjusting my food to the recommendations these videos were suggesting. It did not take long before I started feeling even better. I also watched Youtube videos and anything else I could get my hands on around healthy eating, emotional eating and exercise. The more knowledgeable I became and the more I put it into action the more success I had as the weeks went on.

It is likely that old feelings start creeping up in Week Two. The excitement of starting has likely waned off a bit and cravings and old feelings are likely calling your name. Getting through this time successfully will likely help determine if you are going to have longer term success. So hang in there! I used my supports to check in with as I started to want to give up a bit in week two.

The excitement wasn't there so much and I felt a little scared that I would either fail or never be able to eat junk food again.

As stated earlier, to help me stay motivated, I listened to motivational speakers on Youtube There are lots of different videos to choose from. I found music with a beat to it that was combined with motivational speeches worked really well for me. As I worked out I found my beliefs regarding hard work, integrity and not giving up become stronger. I was inspired by the stories of others and how if I kept moving forward I would achieve my goals and become my own champion. It was an exciting thought and I envisioned myself being strong, lean and powerful. I began to start saying affirmations to myself in week two and the more I said it the more I believed it.

At the end of week two I had another treat day which caused me to gain a few pounds but again I took it off quickly. I stayed true to my commitment to eating healthy the next day which was challenging as my body and mind were telling me they wanted more sugar and processed food. I had to fight these cravings and look at the bigger picture of what I wanted to achieve. I also thought about the consequences of eating unhealthily for a few more days. I would likely fall off for good and begin the old cycle of eating, depression and weight gain. I was determined to not let this happened which I continue to be grateful for today.

Week 3

In week three I began having headaches, upset stomach and low energy and mood. For some people this starts earlier in their weight loss journey. What I realized was I was likely detoxing from a diet of sugar and processed food. I told myself that, like cravings, this too shall pass. And it did. I also decided to wean off soda pop and as I did this, pop started tasting more chemical and artificial to me. At one time I thought pop gave me a boost when in actual fact it was likely leading me down a path of possible health issues.

My weight loss was steady and I continued to lose weight. Making fine adjustments to my eating helped me continue to lose. I sent my eating journal to my dietician and she was able to help tweak it so it was nutritionally complete while helping me with my weight loss. Exercise continued to be difficult at times but I kept pushing and committed to riding my exercise bike at home and walking. I was getting results already and able to push myself that little bit more. There were also days where I felt upset at myself for letting my weight get back to almost 400 pounds. I had to fight the urge to beat myself up and use where I was at as a reason to just give up. The two voices in my head continued to battle each other, one saying you're no good and the other telling me how proud they were and that I was on the verge of a breakthrough in my mind and body. I kept saying to myself, "Stay the course, trust the process and don't let anything stop you." By doing this I kept the negative thoughts and emotions at bay and if they did rise to the top I did not let them stay there for very long. I kept doing this for the next few months and I believe that by doing the work and giving myself positive messages that I was able to lose 130 pounds by the summer. Yes, exercise and healthy eating were also key but if I hadn't worked through my emotional issues and thinking I likely would have not been as successful as I was.

Week 4

By week four I was able to start seeing a difference in my appearance and outlook on life. As mentioned before, I had a few challenges come up around food and old feelings but I pushed through. I was getting some positive attention and encourage- ment and I began sharing what I was doing. I was sensing a shift in my thinking and feeling more positive. I wasn't so hard on myself and I used my supports - wife, nutritionist, friends, co- workers etc. to continue to work through struggles and receive the encouragement I needed. I didn't push the pace but was happy to have any type of weight loss; one pound or 10 it didn't matter as much as that I was going in the right direction. I also made more adjustments to my exercise and diet at this time, as you will likely have to as well. As I stated before, I stopped

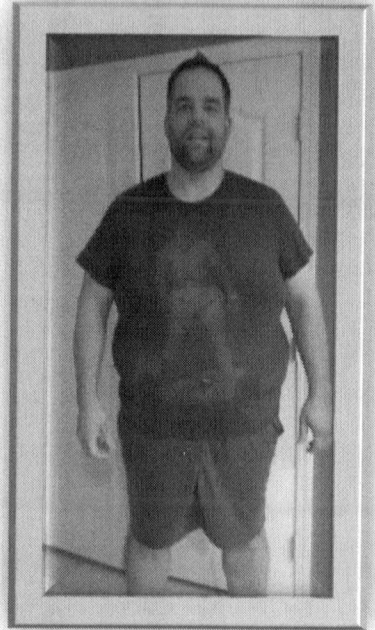

drinking pop. I found that pop didn't give me the energy and healthy feeling that lemon water and power foods did.

For some of you, week four may be really tough. You may not have come as far as you had hoped and are struggling with the inner dialogue telling you that you're not worthy of the gifts you're giving yourself. If you are stuck or have gone back to old ways of unhealthy thinking and eating, then go back to the beginning of the book; refer to earlier chapters including "Am I Ready" and "What I Need To Do To Be Ready." Review the lists you created earlier. DO NOT beat yourself up. Review your story including right up to now and look at your themes. There may be new themes or emotions that have emerged. Again, use your counsellor, friends and supports to work through these feelings while you get back on track. Create new behaviours like phoning friends, going for a walk, drinking water, whatever you need to do to replace old habits of overeating. This may take a few tries, and this is okay as this may be new territory to you. This pattern may be a lifelong process and this is okay. Life is about learning, growing, gaining wisdom and enlightenment. It can be a self discovery journey that is sometimes difficult and sometimes magical. By seeing what is good in myself and others, I have gained a sense of gratitude and appreciation. I began to realize that my past didn't own me. Neither did my old messages about my worth and relationship with food. I had the choice within me to decide what my life would be and I was no longer letting the past dictate my behaviour. This was truly an empowering moment for me but not without its challenges.

Like week three, I also had days in week four where I wanted to give up and fall back into eating junk food. I would tell my wife how much I wanted to eat and hold on to old feelings. I pushed myself to eat healthy at those times and felt better afterwards. I would sometimes go to bed early in order not to eat. The next day I felt great for not giving into negative self messages but for making the choice to take care of me. I also started feeling a shift where my body and mind were beginning to crave exercise and healthy foods. This was different as my cravings usually centered around junk food.

I did have a bit of a bump in the road when I ate too much during my Super Bowl Party. In past years, if I ate or drank too much at Super Bowl, I let myself go back to overeating. But this time in my weight loss journey, it was different. I refused to fully fall. I picked my socks up the next day and truly forgave myself for the unhealthy choices I had made. I had a plan to have some treats but I took it too far and binged on junk food. I had to say to myself that I did what I did but I also had a decision to make. I would either go down the path again of self-hatred and despair or go back to healthy eating. This was really difficult as the sugar and processed food really impacted my thoughts, feelings and overall outlook on life. In just a day or two I went from being optimistic to really negative. My wife and I could really see how food impacted me, not only in my weight gain but emotionally. In a month I had already learned many lessons. I would end up having to go through these lessons a few times until I truly got them. But once I did I felt unstoppable.

Chapter 10

Hitting Your Stride

Weeks 5-8

By week 8 I was down over 40 pounds. I tend to lose weight quite quickly and your weight loss may be different. Remember, this is a journey and not a race. If you lost 10 pounds or 60 by week six, it's all good. You may choose to celebrate in a healthy way by having friends over, going out on a date, going on a small trip or by purchasing something you have been wanting to get. It doesn't matter if you have 20 more pounds or 150 pounds to go; you're going in the right direction, so be proud.

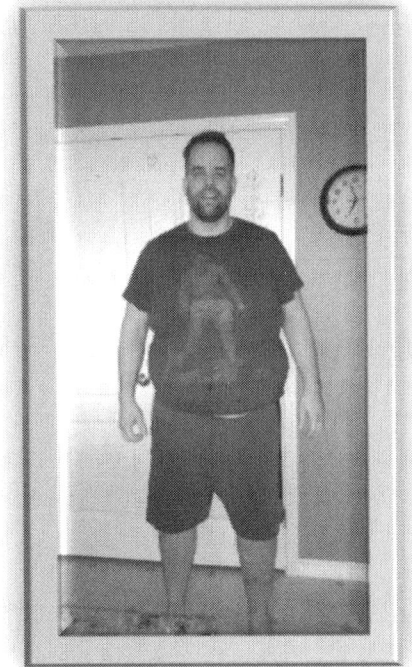

Also note that if you have lost very little or none by this point, then you need to re-evaluate your eating plan and exercise routine. Make adjustments and ask for help from your health professionals to tweak your diet. I have found that I could exercise all day but if my eating plan was off I still gained weight no matter how much I exercised. I was fooling myself in thinking that I could lose weight by just exercising for two hours. As I mentioned before, I could eat healthily and still lose weight but, without exercise, losing weight was much slower and I didn't feel as good.

As you can see, I believe that weight loss and weight management is 95% related to the emotional work and once you have your thinking right, your behaviours will change too. Making healthy eating choices and exercising 5-6 times a week will become a habit and a part of who you are. A transformation will take place and people will begin seeing you differently. The trick is to see yourself differently too.

It is my hope by weeks 5-8 that you have created some new habits and coping techniques that come more naturally and aren't forced. Staying committed at this time is huge. At about week 6, I went back to my gym and incorporated weightlifting with my cardio. Weight Lifting is fun and a great way to build muscle, core strength and keep you looking young. It also aids in weight loss, especially if you remember to incorporate leg workouts. Your biggest muscles and calorie burning opportunity lie in your legs and not in your smaller arms.

As I lost more weight, I began getting lots of attention and people were cheering me on and telling me how well I was doing. In the past, I would have minimized their compliments and brought attention to something I was struggling with or not achieving. This time I just said thank you and smiled. I took in the praise and felt good about myself. I didn't listen to my inner voice saying things like, "Yeah you lost lots of weight but you gained a pound in week 7." I found that when I took a step back and looked at the bigger picture, I already had come a long way. I had met some of my short term goals with weight loss and the change in my thinking. I needed to be proud of this and continue to say, "Way to go Daryl! You rock!"

As I entered week 9 I felt like I had lots of momentum behind me. I also found the negative thoughts had less impact. By being consistent, continually challenging myself to up my game, both physically and emotionally, as well as making good food choices, I began feeling unstoppable. I continued with the positive self messaging, educating myself on nutrition and whatever else I could get my hands on related to weight loss.

I also continued to lose weight with some temporary weight gains after a treat meal or day. These days did slow down my progress but I was also able to enjoy a nice meal with friends and still lower the number on the scale. Tough days continued to come and go but my resolve and overall progress did not stop. I actually began fearing what would happen if I gave up and began overeating again. This was different for me as I had been cocky in my past weight loss attempts. I realized that if I got cocky this time, and did not train, I would likely become complacent and start gaining weight again. Like a champion who becomes lazy, the chance that they will lose their title is much greater if they choose not to train every day. Yes, we need breaks, and I gave myself some. But I also did not stop doing the work to be successful. You need to be your own champion and train even when you don't want to, fight food addiction when it calls your name and never let your guard down as food and negative emotions will easily slide back and knock you on your butt.

Week 9-16

Through weeks 9-16, I continued to adjust my diet and increase my exercise intensity. I also continued to gain more knowledge about healthy power foods, exercise and positive thinking. There was no end to my interest in health and exercise. I wanted to learn everything I could. I journaled my weight loss and how I felt. I continued to be cognizant of old patterns and the consequences of them when I wanted to slip into old behaviours. I forgave myself when I made unhealthy choices. I didn't let unhealthy choices go on for days but got right back on track. I began discovering how tough and powerful I truly was becoming.

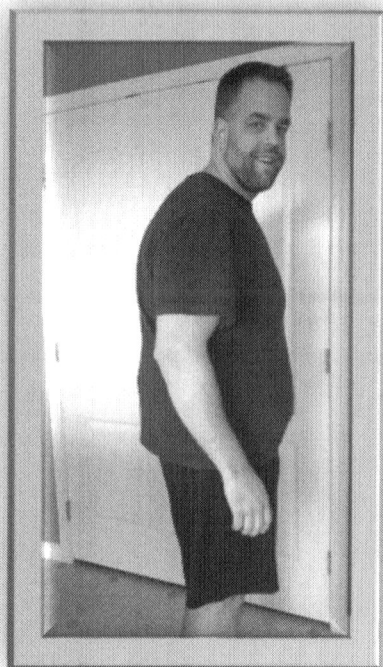

Many people saw the weight I had lost as well as my overall change in attitude towards life. Many of them started asking me about health, exercise and weight loss. I could see who was genuinely interested and who was just looking for a magic answer. When people heard that it took discipline, making tough choices when times were hard, and that they would also need to look at themselves emotionally, they either changed the topic or glazed over. A lot of people thought I would tell them about a magic diet or exercise that they could do quickly with limited effort. When I said this wasn't the case, I could see their disappointment. This made me realize that I could either go back to being stuck like them (those not really interested in doing the work) or continue on my journey to successful weight loss. More than ever I was resolved to never go back to a life of food addiction.

I also wasn't waiting to be at my goal weight to start celebrating the smaller goals I was achieving. I realized I needed to be living in the now and not wait until I was fifty or a hundred pounds lighter to celebrate and do the things I wanted to. I had been waiting my entire life to be thin so I could do and be what I wanted. I saw that there were times that I was existing but not truly living. Junk food had been clouding my mind. When I realized that food was keeping me in a dark place emotionally, I committed myself more than ever to my journey. I started appreciating the big and small things in my life including the interactions with those around me. All my different experiences (playing in the park with my kids, date nights with my wife, hanging out with friends) were so much richer because I was connected to the present and my mind was clear. Food had been pleasurable at times but I started seeing that taking in nature, exercising, and, most importantly, really choosing to love the people in my life gave me even more pleasure. No amount of food could add up to the pride and joy that I was experiencing. Life began feeling like it should and this excited me even more. However, what I did not realize was that, on the horizon was one of the biggest challenges that I would need to face in my weight loss journey. This challenge would either set me back months or I could take it as a learning opportunity. I needed to put into action the commitment and plan I had made for facing a roadblock in the way of my goals.

By week 16 I was down about 70 pounds and I was feeling great. Workouts were going well and I was looking to the next level of fitness. I could see myself in the future getting back down to my goal weight and doing events like Tough Mudder or a half marathon. Then, on April 22, 2015, I was rear ended on my way home from work. After the initial impact, my first thought was, "If I'm really hurt then what will happen to my weight loss journey?" I resisted the negative thoughts in my head like, *Here we go again – I'm finally having some success and now I won't be able to finish.* I said to myself that I would find a way to keep my journey going. I thought about all the work I had done around facing challenges and changing how I responded to them. In the past, this was where I probably would have given up and let the weight go back on. I realized I was faced with a choice – let the accident stop my journey or find a way to take on the new challenge ahead of me.

I decided not to give up and I continue to be grateful for the choice I made that day. I started by getting myself to physio/chiropractor. I was surprised by the chiropractor telling me that I shouldn't stop exercising but that I just needed to slow down a bit and adjust my routine. I also did certain exercises and stretches to help me recover and I continued to keep my eating clean. I was able to make a full recovery in a few months and continued to lose weight. I believe that I was able to do this because of the changes I had made in my thinking and that I made the choice to not fall back into old patterns. I also used my support system and incorporated my chiropractor as one of them as well.

You too may get injured or sick or face some type of emotional challenge. Remember that this will be the most vital time to put your new tools into action. As you know, unhealthy food won't fix the challenges put in front of you. Choosing to use the tools in your arsenal, including eating a healthy diet, finding a way to exercise around an injury and utilizing the emotional support you need will help you prevail. Now I know that if I'm hurt again I have the skills and support to work through it. This knowledge also gives me some reassurance and it is empowering, especially in those times of uncertainty or emotional upheaval.

Weeks 17-25

By week 20 I was about two-thirds of the way to my goal weight. I was getting lots of compliments and people continued to ask me how I was losing the weight. I was down to about 319 pounds and wondering how I was going to do the final push to reaching my goal weight.

A friend spoke to me about a weight loss challenge group to help give me more motivation. Training partners, weight loss groups, personal trainers, running or crossfit groups are all different ways to help motivate and keep you accountable. You may want to

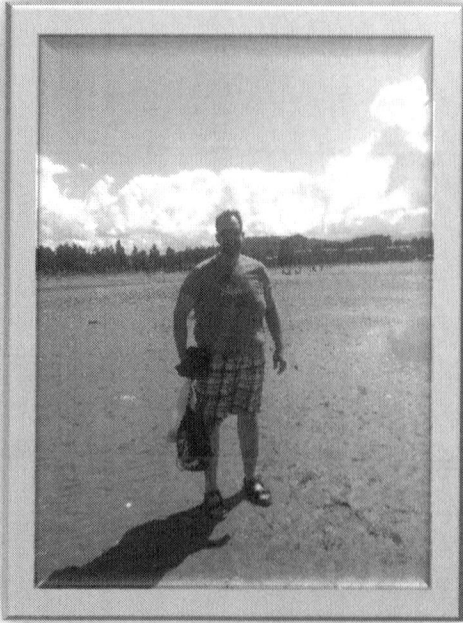

start with a group right away, or later on like I did. The groups aren't for everyone but if you're interested in trying one, I say go for it. When people feel accountable to others they tend to be more motivated to stay on track. You need to be accountable to yourself first. There is a danger that when you leave the group and the pressure is off, you may lose the motivation to keep going on your own journey. I recommend using a group as a support to your journey but not for the reason to keep you going. Groups will come and go but your journey is for life. So, knowing how to stay motivated and moving forward is imperative to your ongoing success.

I ended up joining the weight loss challenge group and winning the challenge. I enjoyed the support, the weigh-ins and the accountability it gave me. The group also gave me the added push to lose another 46 pounds and by July 2015 I was 260 pounds – 20 pounds away from my goal weight. I had lost 135 pounds and felt amazing. I was able to run around with my kids, be a better football coach and I had a sense of positivity that felt incredible. I began jogging once a week and climbing the stairs (255 of them) by my house. I could barely do two sets in March but by the summer I was able to get 5 sets in. I started riding my bike again and my strength increased at the gym. Again, there were days that were very challenging, so using my supports and strategies to stay on track helped me with my success.

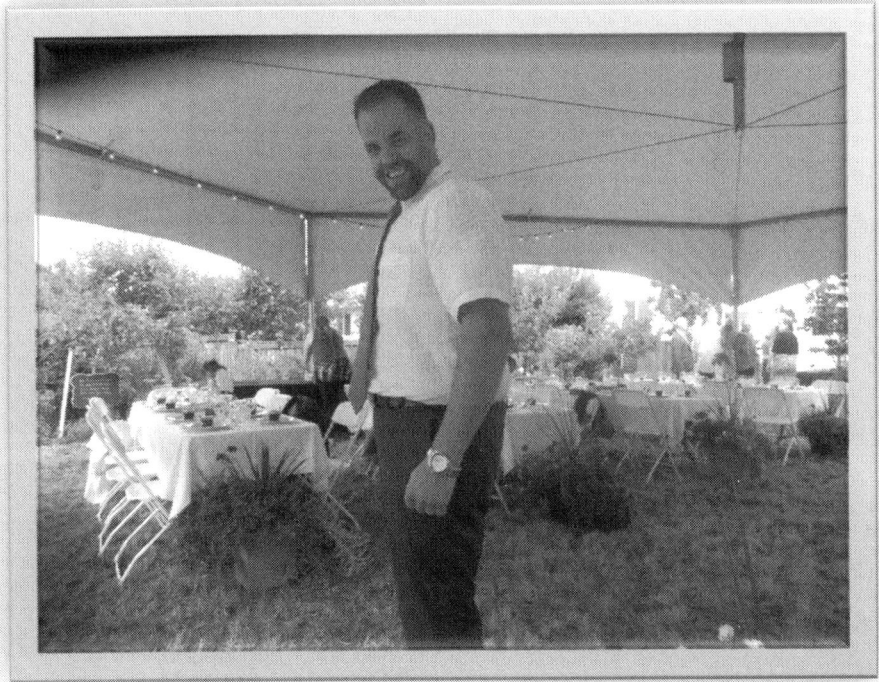

Also, during the summer of 2015, I had 3 weddings and a stag to attend. I was a groomsman in one of the weddings and was really excited to buy myself a suit that I felt good in. I wanted to enjoy all the weddings and the stag but still keep on track with my healthy lifestyle. I did this by ensuring that between the events I ate clean. I knew if I let things go over the summer I would likely have had a major weight gain. I discovered that I could eat well and still have a great time without gaining weight. Yes, I enjoyed the food and some libations but I also didn't let things go too far. I exercised and ate healthily and stayed true to my new way of being.

I also kept challenging myself to do more flights of stairs by the beach where I lived. I rode my bike more, I tried different exercises and increased the amount of weight I was lifting at the gym. I kept on finding new and exciting ways to exercise and keep it fresh. I continued to educate myself about health and exercise and talk to people about my weight loss journey. My cheering section was there for me in both good times and challenging days and my weight continued to come off.

Chapter 11

Going the Distance

Week 26-52

By September 2015, I began thinking more about what the next level looked like for me. I decided it was not only getting the last 20 pounds off but also pushing myself to be in even better shape, both physically and mentally. I made a new friend at my gym who had similar goals and we began working out and pushing each other both in how we worked out and how we thought about life. I adjusted my diet and lowered my calorie intake in order to lose the last 20 pounds, which I did by December 2015. I especially watched my carbohydrate and dairy intake. I increased the intensity and frequency of my workouts and watched how much I ate with my treat meal.

If you find yourself hitting plateaus as you near your goal weight, then you may want to re-evaluate your calorie intake and make adjustments to what you're eating and how much you're exercising. The last 10-20 pounds is often the hardest to lose but it can be done. I'm still working on toning the last little bit of weight but enjoy the challenge. Don't be too hard on yourself and seek support (dietician, personal trainer etc.) if you don't find yourself losing the weight as quickly as you would like.

Also, be careful with how much you eat when you're having a treat meal. As I mentioned before, I would find myself eating too much on my treat meal day and sometimes gorge on the foods that had made me obese and unhealthy in the first place. I needed to start asking myself why I still needed to do this and what payoff binging on really unhealthy food was having when the other six and two third days of the week I ate super clean and healthy. I also had to ask myself if the unhealthy food was helping me feel included and accepted as I usually ate it with friends and family? Was the unhealthy food keeping me from reaching my full potential? What was I afraid of and did I really believe that I was truly deserving of what I dreamed of doing? This strategy (one treat meal or night a week) helped me lose 155 pounds but now I felt it was holding me back.

I began to realize that the choice of really going for my dreams was as big a choice as deciding to get fit/healthy in the first place. I had blamed everyone else in the past for why I was overweight. Once I took responsibility for my choices and decided to act, I saw that I was powerful. I was no longer invisible. I often hear overweight people say that they're big but also invisible. I understand what they're saying as being 400 pounds and 6'3" people noticed me for a second but then I seemed to disappear. The world is a judgmental place and we often base our worth on whether we are noticed and accepted. When we are ignored, we often can start feeling like we don't matter. I found that as I lost weight I became more confident and people noticed me more. It's human nature, so I tried not to be angry about it for long but embraced the attention. So stop being invisible and get out there and fully enjoy life.

I also had to have a talk with myself so that I could begin seeing that I wasn't morbidly obese anymore. I had to spend time looking in the mirror to start accepting the way I looked and the happier feelings I was feeling. Redefining how you see yourself is exciting but sometimes really hard. I needed to stop seeing myself as a 400 pound man. I struggled at times not to see myself this way and realize that I had changed. I allowed myself to be proud and confident and, yes, maybe a little vain at times – ask my wife. I needed to look in the mirror and say, "Daryl this is you now." The little voice trying to pull me back was not as loud but still there at times. I began listening more to the voice that said, "You're fit, smart and powerful. And you can do or be whoever you want to be." I started giving myself more positive messages and saying out loud what I wanted. I saw the effectiveness of this, as I was a successful applicant for a supervisor job I had been trying to get for 5 years and I began writing this book.

It wasn't always an easy path to my success. I encountered those who supported me and those who wanted to bring me down. I learned that true friends want you to reach your full potential. If someone isn't encouraging you or supporting you, then maybe you need to reevaluate your friendship or at least create some space away from them. I'm not saying to drop everybody who is negative about your life change but also be cautious that too much time with them may pull you from the new life you're living. By sticking to your dreams and goals, you may inspire those who have lost hope. So find that balance and remember this is your life to live. Accepting mediocrity and allowing yourself to be held back is not part of reaching your potential.

I also started giving back. My gym asked me to do before and after pictures for their Facebook page. At New Year's, the local news did a TV story on my weight loss journey. I had over 70,000 views and 700 likes. People messaged me on Facebook about my journey and I even met with a few of them in person. I spoke to my mother's weight loss group and got an amazing reception. I realized that I needed to share my story and help anyone that wanted to listen. It's amazing and so rewarding! And you can do it too. I will admit that I struggled to allow myself to enjoy my success at times as I worried it would fall apart. But it didn't and I continue to enjoy my life and build my knowledge about diet, exercise and emotional health. Do I still have days that I eat a little too much and then pay for it the next day? Yes. But I have a found a way to make it work and I refuse to listen to the voice telling me to go back to an unhealthy cycle of eating and then feeling guilty.

As I have said, this journey never ends until we take our last breath. Our goals need to be fluid so that when one is met we are already starting the next. Getting to a goal weight is just a small goal in the bigger scheme of things. The next level in health and exercise and inner growth has no limits unless you decide that it does. Never stop growing and looking to the next level. Food is the fuel but what we do out there in the world is living. So, what do you see for yourself in the next year, both with your weight loss as well as getting to that next level? What more do you want from your life?

It doesn't matter if it takes you 9 months or 3 years to get to your weight loss goal. It's your journey, so enjoy it! Life will bring you challenges and it will be up to you to decide how you work through them and grow. So stop wasting the valuable time you have on this planet and do what moves you. It's your life to live so go out and live it.

Chapter 12

Getting Real Once and For All – The Final Commitment

In the later stages of writing this book, and after a few read throughs, my wife said to me, "Okay, one more chapter and you're done." I was confused because I thought the book was complete. I decided to think about what she had said. And then it came to me. It was a Saturday at about 11:30 at night and I was lying on the bathroom floor looking up at the sink wondering how I got down there.

It wasn't any different than most Saturday nights except that I had eaten more junk food than usual and felt really sick. I ate until I felt overfull, while at the same time hoping that this was the last time I binged. By 11:20 I was in pain and felt nauseous so I went to the bathroom and was sick (I will save you the scary details). The next thing I knew, I had fainted and was on the bathroom floor looking up at the sink wondering what had happened. It was at this moment in my life I realized what my wife was talking about and that my life was about to change even more.

I still felt the need to eat junk and I often binged once a week. I had made some changes over the year and my trick or hack was to have one treat night a week. The treat night was usually connected to a social event so I could have what I liked and enjoy it. The next day I would usually get right back on track and spend the next few days losing the 5-10 pounds I had gained. During those days, I would find myself in a bit of a depression and not so upbeat about life. I would beat myself up for gaining the weight in one night that I had spent all week to take off. This had worked for me when I wasn't near my goal weight as I could lose what I put on during the weekend fairly quickly and then go on to lose more. I stayed on a steady pace with my weight loss. However, this worked for only so long and then I realized that getting to my true goal weight wasn't going to happen until I made the final commitment.

I thought about how food, for so long, had been my protection and life companion. By choosing not to eat junk food, I felt like I was letting go of my security blanket for good. I worried what others would say and do if I didn't fully succeed and I feared that I would be alone if I chose to eat healthily while others didn't. Some people I knew also tried to sabotage my success. I realize now that they were jealous or, more often, they simply didn't feel good about themselves.

I found myself at a fork in the road. I had some choices to make: choose to binge weekly and not fulfill my goals, turn around and fall back into old eating habits or let go of unhealthy food once and for all. I will admit that it took me time to decide this. I felt like an alcoholic that still got drunk once a week but the rest of the time the world thought I was sober and a non drinker. I would say, "Okay one last binge and then I'm done". But I paid the price the next day by feeling depressed and full of anxiety and worry that I would be heading back to a life of food addiction. I called it my food hangover. It was a vicious cycle. This pattern weighed (pun intended) heavily on me, and for me to fully achieve my potential, I had a choice to make. I had set myself a limit on success that I needed to bust through in order to live the extraordinary life I dreamed of; a life where I could make a difference in the world that I knew deep inside I had the potential to do.

For some reason, I didn't want to fully let go of junk food or having the splurges even though it was weighing on me and I knew this couldn't go on forever. Making the final decision to commit to a life of healthy eating without the junk food binges was really frightening. It was the last thing I needed to do in order to have a life free of food addiction. I knew I no longer wanted to be handcuffed to junk food. But I had to ask myself what need the junk food binges were serving. I then asked myself some more questions. Was I scared of being left out when everyone else was eating cake? Was my need to feel included with others and the food they were eating stronger than my need to feel good on the inside and outside? Was not eating junk going to make me face feelings that I was still able to numb out with food? Was I scared of fulfilling my dreams or being disappointed if things didn't fully work out for me?

I struggled with these questions and feelings for months. I avoided facing these questions until I hit rock bottom and, in my case, this was the bathroom floor.

I chose to go for it and let go. I made the final commitment. Like choosing my start date, I chose a day and stuck to it to no longer binge eat. This was a scary thought for me as it meant letting go of junk food binges that I often found myself daydreaming about mid week. Life had started to be about the Saturday treat night that then turned into the Saturday night binge night which sometimes went into the next day. People saw that I continued to keep the weight off but I was only fooling myself because I had not totally changed my unhealthy eating ways. This doesn't mean that having a gourmet piece of pizza, a steak and salad or something else you enjoy is not okay. But it needs to be in moderation and not every day. On Saturdays I was eating pizza, popcorn, chocolate, cookies, pastries and crackers in a period of just a few hours. I am embarrassed to admit it, but I realize it was part of my healing and you may need to do this too. I thought it was okay as long as I didn't let my weight gain go past 20 pounds before I would exercise and eat healthily to get it off. But, I came to realize that I was still eating like a food addict but just in shorter cycles.

I don't regret making this final commitment in the slightest. Instead, I became even more powerful, even when myself and others told me I couldn't do it. I stopped listening to the little voice in my head telling me I couldn't and listened to the voice that said anything was possible. I pushed through and now my book and speaking engagements have brought me to places I never thought possible.

I was moving through the last chapter of my emotional journey to successful weight loss. I was no longer powerless over food and I had control over the choices in my life. Often I heard other people (and sometimes myself) say, "I would eat healthy or I would exercise if it wasn't for..." Well, I'm here to say that as long as we put our past, what people say to us, or our own negative thoughts in the forefront, we are destined to stay at the mercy of our emotions and unhealthy eating. I realized that I am just as worthy as anyone else and deserve a happy life. Food served a different purpose other than to fuel my body for 43 years. But once I decided to fill myself up with self love and relationships/connections, I felt powerful and decided the world was going to be what I wanted it to be.

There are still days that are tough. Sometimes I am tempted to binge eat. But I just take a moment and think of the consequences that overeating will have. I am able to make healthy choices. It takes practice and doing it repeatedly will help create a healthy habit. Food isn't my world now. I can focus on other things that make me happy including my children, wife, extended family, work, hobbies and helping others. It's a fulfilling life that I work on improving everyday and now I work so others can have this life too.

Chapter 13

Weight Issues And Relationships

Whether it is the husband or the wife or both who struggle with emotional eating, the likelihood that food addiction impacts the relationship is very high, especially when one or both of you have weight issues and are not on a healthy eating plan at the same time. If you eat out together, this can get expensive. And if you do it too much, financial issues can start. Also, if one person is trying to lose weight and eat well, and the other is not, resentment may appear from either or both sides. One person may be resentful that the other is not eating well in the home or trying to be healthy. Also, the partner who is losing weight and getting lots of attention may feel resentment from the other who isn't. The partner who is not eating well may try to sabotage (consciously or not) the spouse's success. The spouse who is eating healthily may eventually give in to the temptations around the house and start eating poorly.

My wife and I struggled to be on track together. We would have good intentions at first but then one or both of us would fall off, blaming the other or ourselves. Only recently have we both gotten on track together. If your spouse also struggles with food addiction, it is much more likely that you will both succeed if you are both on the same page and both ready to become healthy, for life.

Being active together, including cooking healthy options and exercising together is a great start. Try to educate one another on what you have learned. Plan your outings away from food and more around an activity that is fun. If you do go out to eat, try making good choices together. Boost one another up. Give each other compliments, especially when goals are reached or you notice physical changes. Also, hold each other accountable but in a supportive and non-controlling way. When one partner is having an unhealthy food choice, you can call them on it but then suggest making a healthy choice later. Sometimes we want to do the opposite of what our partner is telling us to spite them, even if it isn't in our best interests. Remind your partner how far they have come and how good they are looking. This will help him or her get back on track sooner.

If your partner fully falls off the plan, don't join them. You stay the course and continue to encourage your partner to get back on. Be your partner's strength! Support and cheer for them without imposing guilt or shame. If they need to see a counsellor to address emotional issues related to food addiction, maybe go with them to some of the sessions. You may learn where you are actually impeding your spouse's success. You will also likely learn how you can help them and yourself be successful. Often, men and women have different views on addressing issues so talk to your spouse about what is helpful to them when they need support. Good communication and a positive attitude will take you farther in your journey together. There will also be many benefits including a closer emotional connection, more intimacy and you will have more fun. You will not feel alone in your weight loss journey when you have a supportive friend there for you in good times and bad.

Chapter 14

Weight Loss Issues and Children

Your eating habits will definitely impact your children's health. If your children eat unhealthily with you, they will need support in making the change when you make the shift. Going cold turkey, with no snacks, may be too much of a change. Their tastebuds will need to get used to new foods, flavours and textures. Swapping out unhealthy snacks with healthier choices is a great place to start. It will take time but eventually your children will request tasty, healthier choices. Finding a balance between mostly healthy choices and a small treat is your best bet. Including your children in your journey may help get them on board. As they see your healthy choices and changes, they too may want to do the same. Talk about health and exercise often and be positive.

Also, find family activities that provide exercise opportunities and fun such as hiking, playing games, and swimming. Whatever it is, have fun with it! I help to coach both of my sons' football teams which helps me stay active with them.

It's important to also help your kids with the emotional part of eating by talking to them about their feelings and finding healthy ways to cope with problems, rather than numbing those feelings with food. Role modeling healthy eating and exercise is the beginning of the process. Make positive affirmations towards them and encourage them to think and speak positively about themselves. Reassure them that you have their backs, which will also help them feel supported and help to build their self-esteem. You could also have them read this book, or parts of it, to help them see their story, pattern and themes around food. Discuss with them different behaviours and rewards as well as looking at food in a different way. This dialogue will help your child shift away from overeating. Help them see that food is fuel and that they can still enjoy treats with friends but need to be mindful of how much and what they are eating.

Building your child's self esteem and working with them around their feelings with food will help your child start making different choices. Shaming, blaming or talking to them when they are not eating well will likely not work. Get active with your child and make healthy and good tasting meals together. Walks, runs, sports (whatever activity they enjoy) and doing it together will help your child feel that they are not alone in this and that there is a different way of being that they can enjoy.

Finally, some government health departments have programs for children and/or families with weight challenges that may be worth looking into. Counselling around food, emotional and family issues for your child and yourself may also be a tool in addressing overeating. Avoid drastic changes. Slow and steady changes will likely cause less of a rebellion in your home. Sometimes a child just maintaining their weight as they grow taller will be enough to help them reach a healthy size. Learning healthy ways of coping and eating now will help your child have a healthy lifestyle for the future.

Chapter 15

Alternative Weight Loss Options (Surgery)

For some people, change in diet, exercise levels and working through the emotional challenges of weight loss is not enough. Like myself, my wife has struggled with her weight. For her, surgery was an option that she researched and followed through with. Alicia still did the emotional work by seeing a counsellor about her past and present relationship with food. She also educated herself about the surgery, how she would need to change how she ate and how to avoid falling back into overeating behaviours. She has now lost over a hundred pounds and is the happiest I have ever seen her. Our relationship is the best it has ever been and we're both looking to the next level in what we see life becoming for ourselves and our family. I asked Alicia to write about her experience as this may also be an option for you. Surgery is not for everyone. No matter what path you take, going on your emotional journey regarding food and weight loss is needed. Here is what Alicia had to say...

I wasn't always FAT. I was chubby. I was a bit bigger than the other kids my age. But I was never FAT. Until one day I was. At 37 years old I topped the scale at 321 pounds on a 5'3" frame. I looked like a circle with legs. My face touched my chest and there was no neck to be seen. I knew it had to change for me. Life was getting too hard for me and I wasn't even 40 years old. My 60 year old mother had more stamina and agility than I did. I had heard about weight loss surgery and I knew it was what I was looking for.

I booked an appointment with my family doctor to get a referral to the specialist in weight loss surgery. A few months later, there I was in his office learning all about what the VSG (Vertical Sleeve Gastrectomy) could do for me. My specialist had a list of things that I needed to do as his patient in order to get the surgery: things like getting tested for sleep apnea, seeing an internal medicine specialist, checking if I had any hernias, getting my heart tested etc. From the time of my first meeting with my surgeon to the day of my surgery was over 18 months.

It is by no means a quick fix to have weight loss surgery. I believe that this is a blessing because it gives you a chance to both physically and mentally prepare for this new life that you are about to embark on. One of the first things that my surgeon told me to do was to lose weight. I had to prove to him that I wanted this surgery and that I was willing to show him that by losing weight.

The next time that I went to check in with him about how things were going I had gained weight. What? I was so gung ho at first and then I started to get scared and resorted back to old habits of eating away my emotions and feelings. My surgeon gave me the tough love I needed and looked me straight in the eyes and said "If you are not going to work for me, I will not work for you." Thank you Dr. Amson for those words, they were hard to take but they were exactly what I needed to hear.

At my next visit with him I had lost 10% of my body weight. He was so happy and he even put his hand on my shoulder and said, "I knew you could do it". A few short months later I got the phone call that my surgery would be in November. I was so excited and scared all at the same time. And again I resorted back to my old ways of eating away my feelings and had gained back some of the weight that I had lost.

It was getting closer and closer to my surgery and I knew that it was time to get myself mentally prepared for this, which I believe is harder than the weight loss itself. I knew I had to get prepared for a new life and a new way of living without food as my emotional crutch. I knew I had to be ok with the frustration of my life not being what it used to be surrounding food. I had to learn to accept that I would be living a different life now and that going backwards was no longer an option. Most importantly I had to remind myself that I was worth this surgery. I was worth having a better life without my weight holding me back. Once I got to this place mentally, I was unstoppable.

In preparation for the surgery, one month prior, I needed to go on a 30 day liquid diet. What this does is shrink the liver. I did it. I made it the thirty days on only protein drinks and liquids. I was proud of myself for this accomplishment. I had set my mind to it and I did it. In those 30 days I lost 32 pounds. This was a great way to start my new life after the surgery.

The surgery itself wasn't that bad at all. It was less than 2 hours and then I was in recovery. I walked right away and got all the gas out of my stomach. There was a bit of discomfort around the incision area but nothing like I had expected. It took awhile to get used to the feeling of always being full and never really feeling hungry. That went away after about 6 months. Now, I feel hungry but the good news is that I feel full so much quicker. There is no more room for overeating. All in all I feel very lucky with how things turned out.

I recovered quite quickly and was able to start enjoying my new life almost immediately because of the emotional preparation that I did before the surgery. I tried to work through many of my issues and learn to resolve them on my own without food as my crutch. I saw a counsellor and learned how to love me for me whether I was Fat or Skinny. I had to put in the work too. I worked for these results just like Dr. Amson had asked me to. This surgery is not going to fix you. That is your job. This surgery is just a tool to help you do that. It is only one small piece of the puzzle.

What is life like now you ask? My life is what I have always wanted it to be. I am doing things I only hoped to do. I just completed my first 5 km Foam Run with my husband. I am 121 pounds down from my largest weight and still losing. I have gone from a size 3/4XL to a size M/L. I can shop in all stores now not just plus size stores. And the one thing that I have wanted more than anything this whole journey was to be able to cross my legs like a lady and I can do that now. I love it. It is a small thing but to me it is the biggest accomplishment of them all.

I feel normal now. I feel like I look like the rest of the world. I feel confident when I leave my house, not like I want to hide in the shadows of everyone else. I hold my head up high and show the world who I really am. For me this surgery has been one of the best things that I have ever done. It has given me back a life I wasn't living. I will forever be grateful to my surgeon and his team for making all my dreams a reality. The VSG has given me life. One that I am now living to the fullest.

Alicia has also written a book about her experience with weight loss surgery. You can find it on Amazon here: http://www.amazon.com/dp/1540399699

Conclusion

The emotional journey to successful weight loss is not a quick fix but a lifelong journey. It's primarily about doing the "emotional work" to achieve ultimate health. I believe that we can educate ourselves about what we need to eat and how to exercise. But until we figure out what's going on on the inside, we will continue to struggle and go down the wrong path. The emotional journey to successful weight loss is about self discovery and reflection regarding your relationship with food. It's about healing your spirit, heart and mind. You've likely realized from reading my book that food addiction is a symptom of our greater inner struggle(s). The journey often begins with getting to the point of wanting to change.

People are often looking for a quick fix and an easy way. The reality is that successful weight loss is about doing the hard work both physically and emotionally. There is no easy answer, however when we change our attitude the pieces will start to fall into place. It is a journey in both understanding ourselves better and changing our behaviours. It's about listening to the inner voice wanting you to do the things to succeed and ignoring the negative voice calling you down.

Like any journey, it's about preparing ourselves first. When I picked my start date and began my journey I put together everything at my disposal to be successful. In a sense I packed my bag with as many items possible to get me to my destination. I not only educated myself on healthy eating and exercise, I also did the emotional work to break down barriers impacting my thinking and overeating behaviours. I secured a dietician to help me with my food choices. I also found counselling to help me look deeper into why I ate and how I thought junk food was serving me.

I changed my thinking around deprivation and found that I was actually depriving myself of a healthy and exciting life when I ate junk food. I gave myself the power of choice so when I said no to something unhealthy it was because I chose to pass not because I was not allowed. Counselling, books, motivational videos, and documentaries all helped me change my thinking about food and about myself. I learned about my relationship with food through writing my life story and how it was connected to food.

I also created a food journal that linked the emotions I was experiencing with what I was eating. I could then go back and review how my emotions impacted my food choices and how I needed to find a way to make different choices. I set goals and decided that in order to avoid falling back into old habits when I reached a goal I was immediately moving to the next goal. I prepared myself for set backs like disappointments or injuries. I had a plan to work around them until I was better. I created a support network and found ways to still enjoy food and social events without losing sight of what I was ultimately working towards. I did not get cocky but actually scared if I thought I was falling off track for too long.

I have shared with you what my weight loss journey looked like over a one year period. I pulled from many of my experiences and shared the ways I was able to still enjoy a "treat" without a major weight gain. I also shared how I became empowered in giving myself back the choice/control of when and what I ate. I encouraged you to have a cheering section and have some distance from those who weren't able to support you or were stuck in their own addiction.

Weight loss is not a straight line and sometimes the journey is really tough, but it's so worth it. You need to be willing to work through challenges that in the past may have derailed your weight loss progress. By doing the work and staying committed, you can transform yourself into what others only dream about.

It is important to challenge yourself to reach the next level in physical and emotional well being so that you always have new goals to strive for. I made my final commitment to a healthy lifestyle when I let go of the need to have a binge once a week. It was so freeing to let go of the need to binge and, by doing so, I was able to become the person I wanted to be and do whatever I dreamed of. I was no longer a prisoner to food and I was being authentic in that I began fully practising what I preached.

It is my hope that this book will help you heal what is holding you back from the life you truly desire and deserve. I also hope you have learned that you are a complete and whole person at any weight and that you have the power to change your life. By staying committed, remaining disciplined and continuing to be consistent in what you need to do, everything will fall into place.

By putting your intentions out into the world and following through on them (even if the world throws a few road blocks in the way), you will likely create the rewarding life you have always wanted.

I also hope that you see that the next level of fitness and enlightenment is at your fingertips. Striving towards your next goal will help you live a life of unlimited potential and fulfillment. Remember that you are just as worthy of an amazing life as anyone else. When we are overweight and unhappy, this is a hard concept to believe. I am living proof that we can create an amazing life and bust through our own inner adversity. Again, by using your supports, going to therapy, educating yourself on food and exercise and constantly pushing forward, you will find the right path to successful weight loss.

I hope that you have realized that by having self love and being okay with not being "perfect" is actually closer to perfection than trying to be what society tells us is ideal. Embracing your flaws will allow you to stop obsessing over what you're not but, instead, will help you to focus on and love who you really are.

As I have said, your life story is not predetermined and doesn't have to be a sad story. Rather, you can make it a story of perseverance and victory. Looking deeper into why you have gone through what you have and what lessons and gifts have come from it, will help you heal and gain strength and resilience. You may see that your struggle was not for nothing but was necessary for you to heal something within you so that you now can do something even greater in your life. You're not handcuffed to your past or by what anyone said or told you. You decided who you are and what you want from life. It's about letting go of the past and taking action. By working on yourself every day, even in the smallest way, you will be able to continue on the path to successful and maintained weight loss.

In closing, writing this book has been a journey in itself. Looking at my own story and having a hard look at the impact that emotional eating/food addiction has had on me wasn't easy. It was upsetting at times. However, I have realized that my journey has made me who I am today and has shown me that what I have experienced in my life (good and bad) has given me greater inner power. As you read at the beginning of the book, a friend told me that I was chosen for this path because I had the strength to get through it. My journey was actually a gift that I can now share to help others heal and live their best life. So, thank you for allowing me to share my story and be a part of yours. I hope that you have had the chance to make some positive changes and now you too can pay it forward to others with similar struggles. We are no longer alone in our struggle with overeating. As we support each other, we can begin to move out of the clutches of food addiction and into a life full of possibility.

Acknowledgements

Alicia Hill-Marceau - Alicia thank you for pushing me to finish this book and being there for me over the last 20 years. Also thank you for watching the boys all those nights and days when I was writing. Your belief in me helped me fulfill my dreams of sharing my experience and helping others. You're amazing, beautiful and one of a kind.

Lucas and Reid Marceau - thanks for the best sons any parent could ask for. Your humour and encouragement kept me going during the days that I didn't feel like writing.

Douglas and Margaret Marceau - I'm truly blessed to have parents like you. Your excitement and support have helped me stay motivated to finish what I set out to do.

Keith and Robyn Hill - Thank you for always being a support to me, Alicia and the boys. Also thank you for your encouragement and the wisdom you continue to share.

Alison Goliath - Editor - Thanks for cheering me on every step of the way during my journey. Also thank you for the many hours of typing out the book and being honest with me even when it was sometimes not the easiest thing to do.

Shaula Croome – Editor - Thank you Shaula for your excellent editing, ideas and support. The book really took its final shape thanks to you.

Bryan Landry, Craig Gooding, Marc Norris, Andy Lyons and Jeff Houde. Thanks for being my best buddies for over 30 years. I can't say enough how much I appreciate your ongoing support and friendship.

Kevin Perry - Thank you for helping me see the potential I possess and pushing me to go to the next level with my fitness and inner growth.

Amy Yiu - Dietician - Thank you Amy for all those great phone calls and support during my weight loss journey.

Ward Wamboldt - Thanks for all the great Westwood Lake walks and never letting me be a victim in my story. Also thank you for helping me see the brighter side of life and how to be grateful for all things big and small.

Leo, Joanne, Bart, Susan and the other gym staff over the last 9 years. Thanks for all the support and encouragement each day I came into your gyms.

Doug McCrae - Computer tech - Thanks for all your help with our new computer. Having the right equipment made writing a lot easier.

Pierre Trépanier – thank you for all help with our website and marketing.

Suzanne Doyle-Ingram – Publisher – Big thank you to Suzanne for all your support and expertise in turning this book into a reality.

Appendix 1

Eating Plan Ideas

Start with water with lemon to help flush your system. Drink lots of water and if you drink coffee limit the amount of cream and sweetener you use.

BREAKFAST: 2 eggs, onion, peppers, mushrooms and any other veggies you enjoy. I like to add turmeric, pepper, garlic powder, ginger, cayenne pepper as well. I use coconut oil to cook with. Tomatoes, sauerkraut, and half an avocado are also added to my plate.

I also make my own ancient grain hot cereal. I like to go to the health food store and pick out different grains to try. I also add blueberries, cinnamon, NutraCleanse (NutraCleanse includes flax seed, dandelion and other ingredients), hemp seed, and chia seeds to my cereal.

*Because I still weigh 240 pounds and I'm active I like to eat a large breakfast. These foods give me a rush and I feel full, powerful and energized for the day. Google superfoods or go to your local health food store and talk to your local health professional about these foods.

SNACK: banana. Kefir yogurt with local honey and cinnamon added.

LUNCH: I like to have a turkey, bean chili with veggies added. Another option is having leftovers from dinner including chicken, fish, turkey and raw or cooked veggies or a salad.

SNACK: orange, apple or other fruit and trail mix. I make my own trail mix up by going to the health food store and picking out different nuts, seeds, cacao nibs. I only have a small handful as there are a lot of calories in my mix.

SUPPER: turkey, chicken, fish (once a week), chili, beef stew, cut up veggies, steamed or baked veggies or a large salad with kale, spinach, tomatoes, celery, peppers, cauliflower, broccoli, you name it. I limit the amount of dressing I use.

SNACK: I try not to eat after 8 PM. I usually have a piece of cheese and a small piece of dark chocolate. I like to drink tea sometimes or kombucha. Kombucha like kefir, yogurt and sauerkraut are fermented foods with billions of probiotics for digestive health.

FOODS I AVOID: Bread, pastries, baked potatoes, processed foods - especially those with flour and sugar. I don't drink pop and alcohol is limited to the odd drink.

I don't eat a lot of red meat. Red meat has been linked to possible health issues like heart disease so I choose to limit how much of it I eat. I'm working towards less meat and dairy overall in my eating plan and more towards a plant based diet. There appears to be a growing amount of evidence in regards to the health benefits of a plant based diet.

I don't avoid healthy fats like avocado and some dairy and oils. It's not so much about no fat but what fat you choose. Again there is lots of information out there so do your homework and choose wisely.

* Remember that if you have a treat try not go crazy and pick a quality treat like fish, steak, gourmet pizza etc. Limit it to that and try not to binge. You can still enjoy food and, as you know, it's about consistent healthy choices.

I hope these food ideas are something you try and like. Remember to consult your doctor or health professional when changing your diet. This is especially important if you have diabetes, heart issues or any other health condition that is impacted by diet.

Appendix 2

Movies You May Want to Check Out on Netflix and Youtube:

- Forks Over Knives

- Food Inc.

- Fat, Sick & Nearly Dead

- Hungry for Change

- Vegucated

- Food Matters

- Food Choices

Youtube is a great source. I suggest you go onto Youtube and search food documentaries, healthy eating, food addiction, emotional eating, and motivational speeches with music. I also Googled Les Brown, Tony Robbins, Eric Robbins and other motivational speakers to help me stay on track. There is so much out there so have fun and keep educating yourself.

Also there are many great books on diet and exercise. Look for ideas and reviews of books that may also support you on your journey. Again, the list is huge so have fun.

Here are a few Youtube videos I would recommend:

Ted Talk - The Power of Vulnerability by Brené Brown

Conquer – 1 Hour Long Workout with Motivational Speech

Why Do We Fail – Motivational Videos

Best Motivational Speeches Compilation

Tony Robbins – Creating Unstoppable Self Confidence

Tony Robbins – Top 10 Rules for Successes

Tony Robbins – Power of Choice

Jim Rohn – The Greatest Motivational Speech from Jim Rohn

Less Brown – How to Change Mindset

Wayne Dyer – Your Thoughts are Your Reality

Eric Thomas – Secrets to Success

Keep in Touch

Daryl and his wife Alicia have a website dedicated to helping others in their weight loss journey. You can keep in touch with them at www.marceaubooks.com.